"In *Mornings with L
ordinary life and ren
author, friend and fe
of the story with the same sensitivity and thoughtfulness that he
showed in helping take care of Larry in his last days. The result is
a book that captures a man whose life leaves us not with grief,
although that's unavoidable, but with hope that God is stronger
than anything life can throw at us. I knew Larry Browning a little,
but Tom helps me know him a lot—and I finished the book
feeling privileged for that opportunity."

>—BOB WELCH, author of *American Nightingale*, and
>columnist for Eugene's *The Register-Guard*

"I've had the privilege of knowing both Larry and Tom since their
teenage years. Their journeys were separate until they met later in
life. This is a story of faith, challenge, opportunity and a friendship
that can teach us valuable life lessons. It's an up-close look at Larry's
journey that includes wandering, redemption and victory. We see the
humanity of Larry that is met with a grace that is life-changing. We
also discover through Tom that as you pray for something, *you* might
be the answer to this prayer. In that moment of surprise we see this
story unfold. In Tom's personal and insightful way, welcome to this
journey!"

>—RON SAUER, Young Life Regional Training
>Director, Oregon Cascades Region

Mornings with Larry

Mornings with Larry

୫୦ଓୡ

Life Lessons from a
Man in a Wheelchair

Tom Nash

Mornings with Larry
Published by CreateSpace an Amazon company
Copyright © 2018 by Tom Nash

ISBN-13: 978-1545245682

IN MEMORY OF

MY MOTHER, BETTY,

AND MY SISTER, PATTI

CONTENTS

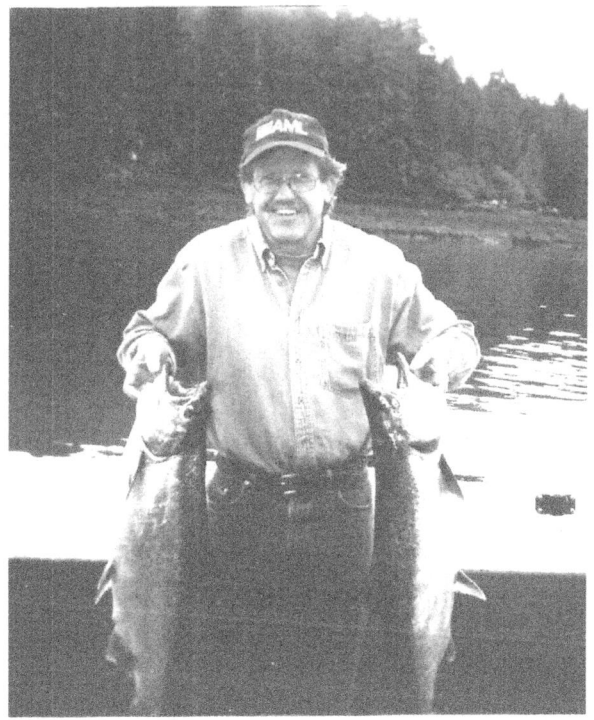

Larry in Wrangle, Alaska, 1999

ACKNOWLEDGEMENTS

I would like to acknowledge Larry's surviving family: his wife Ann, daughter Paige, son Ryan, mother Agatha and sister Brenda. Thanks to Larry's many friends and relatives. Thanks to Bob Welch for loaning me his precious copy of the Tim Ownbey article, *A Soldier Remembered.* Thanks to Pastor Dick Roberts for his amazing Old Testament knowledge, essential for that three-way discussion on the book of Job.

A special thanks to my wife, Denise, who spent hours editing the manuscript—and more hours listening to me drone on and on about the book. Also, she took the striking cover photo of the Persian Ironwood in its autumn splendor.

Finally, I could never thank Larry enough for being a mentor, brother in Christ, pastor, great listener, friend and an incredible role model. And thanks to Larry for his sharp memory, essential for the forty-plus interviews that formed the foundation for this book.

ೞೞೞ

FORWARD BY LARRY BROWNING

"And we know that God causes all things to work together for good to those who love God, to those who are called according to His purpose." Romans 8:28 (NASB)

I was very fortunate as a boy to be raised in a Christian home and taught the truth of God's Word. Although at the age of eighteen I rebelled against God's authority and continued to do so for several years. I've often compared myself to the prodigal son, who when "he came to his senses, returned to his father." In my case, it was not that I came to my senses, but that God brought me to my senses and it was then that I returned to the God of my youth.

After I had returned to Christ and was seeking to live my life for Him, I would ponder how God was going to take the things that I'd experienced in all those years and use them for my good and for His glory.

The first time that I came to understand what God meant by that was when I began working as a part-time chaplain at San Quentin Penitentiary. I was given the responsibility, and I might add, the privilege of ministering to men on death row. At that time I realized that God was using my past rebellious years as a means to be able to share with these men that God can take the vilest things of people and use them for His glory.

Thinking about my past, I realized that I had broken all of God's ten commandments. Often people would ask me, "How can you minister to those men?" I think people tend to forget that God "came to call sinners to repentance," and we are commanded to take the gospel to *all* the world—and that includes San Quentin. People forget that if it were not for God's mercy and grace, they also would be sentenced to death; not only physical death, but spiritual death, which is eternal separation from God. I realized that, yeah, these men had done some very vile things; but at the same time it wasn't because of who I was that God saved me, but it was because of His good pleasure. God had shown throughout scripture that He delighted in taking the most vile and transforming their lives.

Later on, when I began my first pastorate in Dorris, California, I was once again reminded of the reality of Romans 8:28. I saw how God uses all things, the bad as well as the good, to accomplish His purposes. Throughout my twenty years of pastoring, the truth of Romans 8:28 has been confirmed time and time again. Today as I sit in this wheelchair, physically unable to do anything, God continues to show me that He does "work all things together for the good to those who *love Him* and are called according to *His purposes.*"

I pray as you read through the pages of this book that you will be encouraged to know that God does use all things to work together according to His purpose. If you say, "Larry, you don't know my situation," then I'll say, "You're right—but God does." Let me encourage you to take him at his word. You'll never regret it.

Larry Browning
December 2010

Mornings
With Larry

Mornings with Larry

PROLOGUE

South Vietnam, July 18, 1970

Four olive-drab body bags marked the heart of the perimeter. The encampment barely stirred but for a few guards searching the moonlit jungle for shifting shadows.

A boyish private, unable to sleep, crawled from his tent and sat against a tree. He stared, trance-like, at his four fallen comrades. Pfc. James Larry Browning, age twenty, kept this vigil for much of the night.

The camp broke with the light of dawn. The weary, diminished company of thirty-three soldiers packed their tents and gear. Some paused for a bite of rations. Others smoked or drank coffee.

The distant thump of rotor blades echoed in the damp tropical sky. A medevac helicopter appeared over the jungle canopy and descended toward the troops. It touched down in a small landing zone near the fallen soldiers. Several men loaded the dead into the chopper, which quickly lifted off. Browning lit a cigarette and watched the medevac fly away over the tops of palm trees.

The company divided into three platoons and entered a jungle trail. They trekked until midmorning and stopped for a break near the edge of a small clearing.

Browning slipped off his pack and sat next to another private. A sergeant approached the two and gave orders. They nodded and readied their M-16 rifles for guard duty. The pair patrolled along the edge of the jungle and stopped in dense trees and brush, across the clearing from their company.

Another chopper, a Huey, emerged over the treetops. It descended toward the resting company and landed, blowing a storm of dust.

The noise stole nap time from a handful of soldiers. Others continued to chat, snack or smoke, while casting steely-eyed glances at the helicopter.

The rotor blades churned. Two door gunners, one on each side of the craft, aimed mounted M-60 machine guns into the surrounding jungle. A helmeted passenger dressed in clean-and-pressed combat fatigues sat alone in the back. Black eagle insignias decorated his collar, marking him a colonel.

The company's captain strode toward the landed Huey and waited. The colonel stepped out of the craft, hustled away from the whipping blades, and greeted the saluting captain. They conversed; the colonel laughed now and then.

Unseen in the thick undergrowth beyond the far side of the clearing, Browning and the other private stood guard. They peered through leaves and branches at the captain and colonel, about seventy yards away.

While the officers talked near the helicopter, the two lowly sentries conducted a little conference of their own. They whispered intently for a short time and nodded in agreement.

Browning turned and focused his attention on the two men near the chopper. He adjusted his footing.

The Huey's blades pulsed and sliced. Browning shut out the noise and breathed deeply.

He raised his M-16.

His right thumb touched the safety, his forefinger inched toward the trigger. He fine-tuned his aim.

The sights aligned perfectly on the colonel's chest.

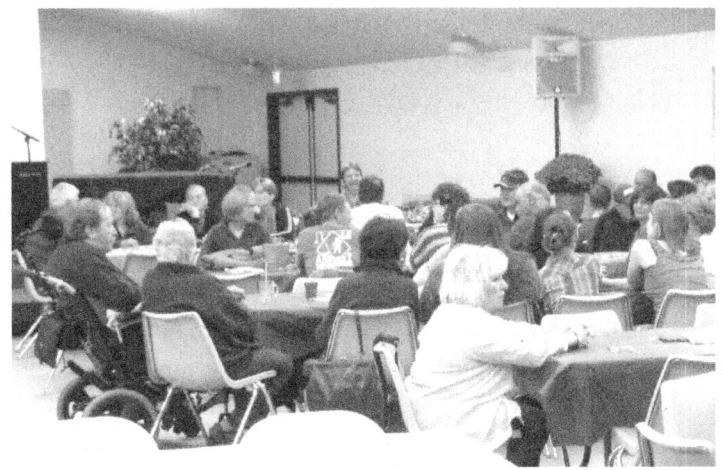

Larry (left) at a McKenzie Bible Fellowship church dinner, 2010

ช०ด

1

SCARED TO MEET YOU, LARRY

The church dinner drew to an end. I swallowed a last bit of carrot cake and glanced past several heads toward the man in the wheelchair. An uncomfortable thought surfaced: *It's about time you introduced yourself.*

I took a deep breath, got up from the table and approached him.

"Hello, Larry," I said, extending my right hand. "I'm Tom. It's good to meet you."

He looked up at me and smiled. "Hi Tom."

His fingers barely moved and his forearm remained fixed on the wheelchair armrest. An awkward moment passed—time enough for me to realize his disability affected more than just his legs. I grasped his limp right hand and shook it for the both of us.

He continued, "I've seen you in church [pause for breath], but haven't had a chance to [pause for breath] talk to you."

Actually, I'd done my best to avoid him, probably due to my shyness and being overly focused on his disability. I had yet to realize Larry's flesh-and-blood human status.

Our first conversation was brief and I was distracted by his frequent mid-sentence pauses for breath. The thought of conversing with a disabled person frostbit my brain. When the encounter ended, I walked back to my seat with a sigh of relief.

If it had been up to me, I'd never have taken our relationship beyond that obligatory greeting. But God sometimes bypasses our unwilling hearts and places us in situations we wouldn't venture to on our own.

That first meeting occurred in 2008 at McKenzie Bible Fellowship in the community of Vida, Oregon. Larry, his wife, Ann, and their teenaged daughter, Paige, had recently joined our church. They soon became fixtures each Sunday morning, claiming three spots in the left front row as their own. Occasionally, their son Ryan took a break from his studies at Oregon State University, ninety minutes away, and traveled home to join them.

Two and a half years earlier, in August of 2005, Larry had resigned his pastorate at Valley Hills Community Church in Springfield, Oregon. The debilitating symptoms of multiple sclerosis (MS) had progressed to the point where he felt he needed to make that hard decision. He describes his condition at that time, "I still had quite a bit of movement in my arms, but no movement in my legs. And I didn't have any problem with my eyes. So I could still preach. But I didn't feel it was fair to the congregation, because most people didn't have wheelchair accessibility [in their homes] and I was kind of a hands-on pastor. So I just felt it was time to step aside and let them call a new pastor who could be more involved."

Some facts about multiple sclerosis:

The National Multiple Sclerosis Society estimates that 2.3 million people worldwide suffer from MS. In the United States, one person out of 750 may develop the disease. Women are at least two to three times more likely to develop MS than men. Nearly half of people with MS suffer from chronic pain. Larry sometimes experiences intense, burning pain that runs from his feet up through his back.

The most common form of MS is relapsing-remitting, known for its ups and downs. Those with this form may lose the use of their legs and then regain use later.

The primary-progressive form, which afflicts Larry, is far less common. It affects about ten percent of those with MS. Decline is steady. Few, if any, remissions can be expected.

MS attacks the fatty myelin sheaths that surround and protect nerve cells. When the myelin is damaged, nerve cells along the spinal cord fail to adequately conduct signals. This results in a variety of debilitating symptoms. When Larry tries to move his legs, the brain's command is stifled before reaching the motor nerves in his leg muscles. Oddly enough, sensory nerves continue to function, so he continues to feel things such as touch, tickles, itching and pain. The cause of MS is still unknown and no cure has been found.

In 2001, Larry was diagnosed with primary-progressive multiple sclerosis, the fast-developing form of the disease. By January of 2008, when I first met him, MS had left him essentially quadriplegic. He could still control the wheelchair toggle with his right hand. His right eye worked fine, but vision in his left eye was blurred.

The Brownings decided they could reduce stress and save time if they attended a church closer to their home. As a result, those of us at McKenzie Bible Fellowship, just three miles from their house, received a great blessing.

Larry preached one Sunday and shared his life story. He'd worn many hats: Vietnam combat soldier, longhaired hippie, preacher, widower, single dad, and modern-day Job. He preferred delivering Bible-based sermons to talking about himself. But speaking opportunities sometimes accompanied requests that he recount his adventurous life and how God brought him to where he is today.

As days went by, the people at McKenzie Bible Fellowship came to know Larry as a friend and brother in Christ. Having put aside his pastoral title, he fellowshipped as one of the flock. As a sheep, he lived out what he'd preached as a shepherd. His conversation typically focused on Christ and others. He didn't complain about his severe disability. It became clear to the new church that he was a man of strong, mature faith.

Larry and Ann began showing up at the same midweek Bible study that my wife Denise and I attended. Before long, the group decided to switch the meetings to the Brownings' home. This gave Ann, a petite woman, a break from the work required to load her husband into the wheelchair van and unload him. The change blessed us all due to Ann's warm hospitality and tastefully decorated home.

One evening, the Brownings presented a prayer request at the Bible study. Larry's morning caregiver, Evan, needed to quit soon. He cared for Larry five mornings per week. Ann cared for her husband Saturday and Sunday mornings, as well as seven afternoons and seven evenings per week. Someone needed to be within earshot of Larry at all times. The Bible-study group prayed for a replacement for Evan.

More than a month passed and the position was still open. The Lord nudged my heart to pursue the job. I felt little enthusiasm. Caregiving? Ugh. The idea made me squeamish. On the other hand, I needed morning work to supplement my plant nursery business. So when I asked Ann and Larry for the job, I did my best to mask these mixed feelings. In July 2009, they hired me—for better or worse.

On day one, Ann introduced me to Evan, my trainer for the next two mornings. That first day, I simply observed him. He began by filling a small plastic container with about a dozen pills and pouring milk into a small glass.

We entered Larry's bedroom, where he lay on his back on a hospital bed, his upper body inclined about forty degrees. He was awake and smiling.

"Morning, boss," said Evan.

"Morning, Evan," said Larry. He looked at me with his still-functional right eye. "How you doing, Tom?"

"Alright, Larry," I said. "How about yourself?" Oops. That was my first mistake. A few weeks later I would learn that it bothers Larry when people greet him with questions such as, "How you doing, brother?", "How's it going?" or, ahem, "How about yourself?" Sometimes he's tempted to give a testy answer, such as, "How do you *think* I'm doing?" However, his verbal responses are always polite.

"Pretty good," he answered me.

The greetings ended and I observed Evan as he performed the seemingly endless tasks required to care for a quadriplegic person. I had no idea all the details involved—and they needed to be done in the correct order. Squeamishness was the least of my worries.

By the end of three hours, Evan and all other caregivers

on planet earth had won my respect. How would my forty-nine year old brain ever remember all this stuff?

On day two, I worked and Evan directed. Sure enough, I remembered little. Evan coached me through the routine, much of which involved learning how to properly move Larry's body. Upon waking, he had to be moved, via a Hoyer (a crane-like lift), from his bed to the shower, then to the wheelchair. After breakfast, he needed to be raised from his wheelchair onto the therapeutic standing frame, where he stood for thirty minutes before being lowered back into the wheelchair. Fighting gravity is not easy.

All this movement meant that poor Larry had to endure this newbie inefficiently shifting/jerking him all over the place. In the middle of it all, he and Evan got into a lighthearted debate over whether or not Larry was dead weight.

"Believe me, boss," said Evan, "you're dead weight."

"Nah," said Larry. "I'm *live* weight."

At the end of day two, I reluctantly said goodbye to Evan and never saw him again. I was on my own.

Evan did great as a trainer, but I wanted a few more days with him. I felt ill-prepared to care for Larry by myself. That night I couldn't sleep. I began day three sleep-deprived, overwhelmed and full of doubts about whether I could do the job.

Fortunately, Larry knew the routine better than anyone, and for the next several weeks he coached me through the sequences, reminding me every time I missed a step. To this day, Larry reminds me when I forget things—such as connecting the urine collection bag to the catheter. You don't want to forget *that*.

More than two years have passed since those first training days, and I'm still a bit scared to see Larry each morning. To encounter him is to be confronted with his hard life, a life that's incomprehensible to those who are healthy. To understand my brother fully would require that I lose the use of my arms, legs—and eyes.

In Larry's words: "Being handicapped is something that—until you've experienced it—you really know little about it. I never would have been able to relate to someone in a wheelchair without having been in one myself. I know people who've spent a day in a wheelchair, and they have discovered the difficulties, but again, it's nothing like being confined to a wheelchair for life, because there is no hope at the end of the day that I'll be able to get out of this."

Most nights, Larry sleeps well, but occasionally he experiences insomnia. Nobody likes to lose sleep, but at least healthy people can toss and turn, get up, perhaps make a snack or read for a while.

Larry likens a sleepless night to being buried alive. "I feel like my body is a casket; I'm inside it and I can't get out."

Certainly there's truth to the saying: "You can't really understand a man until you've walked in his shoes." But in reality, we don't walk in each other's shoes. In every relationship there will be gaps of unknowing mixed with areas of common ground. But even if we can't always relate, sometimes it's just nice to hang out and enjoy each other's mysteries. And Larry has mastered the art of hangin' with people.

When we imagine the difficulties of being severely disabled, the obvious *physical* restrictions come to mind. We couldn't run, walk, throw balls, read, write, watch movies, feed ourselves, blow our nose, fish, hunt, drive, etc. Think of your favorite activities. A blind quadriplegic person probably can't do them, or needs assistance doing them.

I asked Larry what he considered the hardest thing about his condition.

"I think loneliness is probably close to the top," he said.

"It takes away being able to do things with your spouse—like work or sitting on the couch and enjoying watching something together. I'm here by myself because Ann has to keep the yard up, maintain the house, the flowers. So a lot of times I'm just left alone. I sleep a lot, but other times I'm left to listen to the television. Basically, MS has changed the relationship with my wife from being my partner to being my caregiver. And that in itself brings a lot of loneliness."

It surprised me that loneliness would be one of Larry's biggest struggles. It seemed to me the worst thing would be the claustrophobic frustration of not being able to move—that "buried alive" feeling. And Larry does find that awful. But even worse is the isolation he feels from not being able to participate with others in activities that require movement or sight.

"It affects every relationship," he says, "your relationship with your wife, your children, your friends—because all you can do is sit and talk. You can't go down the river and fish, or go for a walk or anything."

Loneliness.

Larry loves fellowship. He describes himself as a people-oriented pastor. His ministry involves relationships, first with God, and then with fellow human beings. Prior to the disease, he led an activity-oriented social life. Whether taking a friend down the river in his drift boat or playing church-league softball, Larry often interwove physical activities with relationships.

But now he just sits. When people visit, he talks and listens.

There are positives in all this. Although Larry detests sitting in a wheelchair twelve hours a day, he enjoys back-and-forth dialogue with others. He has the rare gift of being both a good speaker and a good listener. Larry actually asks me questions about my boring life—and listens to my long answers.

He remembers the names of my nieces and nephews, and knows details about their lives. Now that is something.

"When I interact with other people," he says, "I think less of what I'm going through and instead focus on where they're at. It gives me an opportunity to pray specifically for their needs. Of course, I've always been a people person and I enjoy interaction with people."

He finds conversation even more enjoyable if it involves a road trip. Food and fellowship at restaurants are always a treat for him. We often have breakfast at a local restaurant with a small group of Christian brothers. The camaraderie—and endless refills of coffee—energize him.

I'm glad I stretched myself and telephoned the Brownings on that summer day in 2009. My apprehension was unfounded, and I made an incredible friend. Larry and I talk about nearly everything—whether deep, surface, or over the edge. We've had our share of discussions about theology and Christian life. I suspect he's more candid now than when he wore the pastoral hat. Larry's many past adventures, whether wholesome or unsavory, always involved people and relationships. I'm thankful to play a part in his latest journey.

He's the big brother I never had.

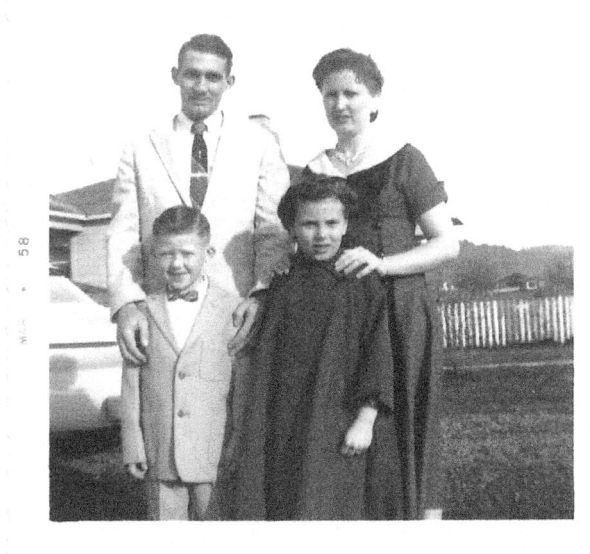

James "Jay" Browning, Agatha, Larry and Brenda, 1958

ଚତ୍ରେଷ

2
DAYS OF YOUTH

It's late in the morning and Larry asks me to check his emails before I leave for the day. The computer is in his bedroom. He directs me to delete most messages, but as usual has me read all prayer requests from his former flock at Valley Hills Community Church. I stifle a yawn and read the requests. To me, they're just names. But Larry listens intently. A young man has lost his job and Larry responds with a "Hmm." A child is very ill and Larry sighs, "Oh." This is Larry's spiritual family. I'm glad I held back that yawn.

I hear the back door open and close. Footsteps echo from the kitchen, then across the hardwood living room floor.

"Hello," says a woman's voice. "Anybody in there?" She speaks in a slow, southern drawl.

Larry's mother, Agatha (pronounced a-GAY-tha) Morse, is here for her weekly visit. I greet her as she enters the bedroom. She smiles at me and turns to her son. "How you doing, hon?"

"Fine, Mom," says Larry. "We're about done."

Though eighty years old, Agatha looks and carries herself like she's fifteen years younger. She's a retired nurse and lives about twenty miles away, in Springfield. A widow twice, her first husband, James William Browning, died in a logging accident in 1970. Her second husband of over thirty years, Lynn Morse, suffered from pancreatic cancer and died in 2008.

We finish with the emails and I wheel Larry into the living room. I adjust the tilt of his wheelchair so he's more reclined. Agatha extends her hands as if she wants to help. It's not the first time she's tried to assist me in my job. One time she inspected Larry's weekly pill organizers to make sure I filled them correctly.

She dotes over her son. The strenuous morning work of getting Larry started is done. Agatha can now spend the afternoon just being with him, performing only a few light-duty tasks to help with his comfort.

"Anything else, boss?" I ask.

"Nope," says Larry. "I'll see you in the morning, brother."

I smile and nod at his mother. "Bye now."

"Bye Tom." She moves close to him.

I leave the living room and head to the kitchen for my keys. Mother and son begin to catch up on news about friends and family. The atmosphere is upbeat and their mutual affection is evident.

I exit the back door and walk toward my pickup. Melancholy thoughts enter my mind—about Larry's frustration at not being able to care for his aging mother, and the heartbreak Agatha must feel as she watches the third man in her life slip away.

&ra;&cb;

A small black and white photograph sits on a shelf in the Browning bathroom. In it, Larry, about age four, leans against the right knee of his dad, James Browning. They pose in front of an open garage door. The father, wearing a white shirt and black tie, is dark-haired, slender and handsome. He allows a hint of a smile. Squinty-eyed little Larry appears bold and energetic, not unlike Dennis the Menace. James' right arm reaches across Larry's back as if to steady his son. A cigarette is visible between the dad's fingers.

Larry remembers an incident that occurred about a year after the photo was taken. He had snuck one of his dad's cigarettes and lit up. James caught him and asked, "What are you doing?" Young Larry answered, "You smoke. Why can't I?"

Larry suspects this was the incident that spurred his father to quit smoking.

Agatha recalls a similar event that occurred in the mid-1950's when Larry was about six. James, or "Jay," as she refers to her late husband, would attend church off and on, but had yet to make a commitment to Christ. One Sunday, Jay decided to skip church. As Larry's older sister Brenda and their mother prepared to leave, Larry pointed at his daddy and said, "If he's not going to church, then I'm not going either." From then on, the father attended church regularly. The next Easter Sunday, Jay invited Jesus Christ to be his Lord and Savior.

Although Larry tested his father at times, he also revered him and loved being around him. Jay's happy-go-lucky personality drew Larry like a magnet. The six year old got a scare once while shadowing his dad. Jay was on the back porch, moving a large ceramic crock of Agatha's homemade pickle relish. The heavy container slipped out of his hands. He tried grabbing it to break the fall, but the crock shattered on the concrete. Jay gashed his hand and blood flowed freely. He passed out before his son's wide eyes.

Larry remembers panicking. "So I go running down the road hollering, 'My daddy's dead! My daddy's dead!' And all the neighbors came back and when they got there, he's sitting in a chair, alive and well."

Larry felt protective toward his father and often waited by the living room window for his dad to return from work. On days Jay came home late, Larry worried about his dad's safety.

When Jay committed his life to Christ, a transformation occurred, evidenced by a major commitment of his time and energy for God and the church. He became a great role model for his son. During the 1950's the Browning family belonged to Trinity Baptist Church in Springfield, where they faithfully attended three times a week: Sunday mornings, Sunday nights and Wednesday evenings. Jay became a hardworking deacon and played key roles in a number of church building projects. He consistently gave up his Saturdays to do volunteer work. Young Larry observed his father to be no passive Christian.

"My dad was very evangelistic," says Larry. "I remember one time I was in my teens, we went to Balboa Raceway [Eugene, Oregon] to watch the drags. Dad said, 'You go ahead and go in and I'll be there in a minute.' And he proceeded to go throughout the parking lot, putting tracts on people's cars. He had a whole drawer full of tracts that he kept and he handed them out all the time."

Larry spent most of his childhood and teenage years in Oregon, but his roots go back to Waynesville, North Carolina, nestled within the Appalachian Mountains, where he was born March 12, 1950. His family struggled financially that year and had no indoor plumbing. Agatha had to carry clothes to a nearby creek and scrub them on a washboard. When Larry was eighteen months old, the family moved across the country to Darrington, Washington. Jay found work there as a logger.

In 1954 the Brownings relocated to Springfield. They moved into a home next to a grade school. At age four, Larry often wandered to the playground during recess and begged his older sister, Brenda, a first grader, to come home and play with him. She usually relented. Her grades suffered and she had to repeat the first grade the next year.

"I was a real good brother," jokes Larry.

During 1961 the Brownings moved back and forth across the country three times. The final trip to North Carolina proved nearly disastrous. A crash outside Albuquerque, New Mexico totaled their car and blew the top off their trailer. Nobody was hurt, but they lacked car insurance. After three days, the family hit the road again in a '56 Chevy sedan that Jay purchased in Albuquerque. Misfortune continued when Jay left his wallet on the trailer hitch. With the wallet and money lost, Agatha cashed the check from the sale of their home in Oregon.

Eventually they arrived in North Carolina, where they lived for the next five years, through Larry's sophomore year of high school. Despite the rough trip getting there, Larry was glad to return to the place of his birth. His best memories involved the time spent with his cousins, rabbit hunting, playing ball or hanging out. He became a good athlete and played all major sports, even making the varsity baseball squad as a ninth grader. His sister, Brenda, became a high school cheerleader. The two siblings loved life in Tar Heel country.

The summer after Larry's sophomore year, the Brownings uprooted one final time and moved back to Springfield, where they settled for good. Jay figured he could earn better income logging in Oregon than working at a tire plant in North Carolina. He enjoyed working in the woods and had never wanted to leave the Beaver State in the first place.

Larry and Brenda hated the move. She had hoped to finish her senior year in North Carolina and Larry had worked hard to earn his stripes as an athlete. In North Carolina, he expected to easily make the varsity basketball team. The Oregon coaches wouldn't know him from Adam. He also hated leaving his best friend, Terry Mease.

Larry attended Thurston High School his junior and senior years. When he first arrived, his Southern drawl drew a fair amount of attention. Some of the girls thought it was cute, but other students teased him. Larry resolved to shed the twang. He soon mastered the flat speech of the West Coast.

He participated in the high school choir and even mustered up courage to sing a solo in a concert. "I was downright scared," he says. He survived and discovered he had pretty good pipes, which would serve him well years later when he formed a Christian rock band.

Larry had developed a passion for hoops while in North Carolina, known for its elite college basketball. But in Oregon he failed to make the cut when he tried out for Thurston's varsity basketball team. This was a significant disappointment. He blamed the coach for showing favoritism toward established players.

"So I became very disenchanted with high school sports and I quit playing. I'd played basketball, baseball, football up until I moved back to Oregon. I never played [school sports] again after that."

Disenchantment would also play a role in his spiritual life. He had become a Christian at age seven, when a pastor visited their home to share the gospel with his sister, Brenda. Larry asked to sit in and listen. He ended up receiving Christ in a tearful conversion. Brenda believed as well.

Larry was baptized on his eighth birthday. His commitment level wavered for the next several years. At age eighteen, he attended a youth revival at Eastside Baptist Church in Springfield. A Texas preacher named Gary Orr gave a message that touched Larry's heart.

"I felt the Holy Spirit speaking to me and I felt that God was calling me into full-time Christian service. I went forward and surrendered to the ministry."

Larry felt called to be a foreign missionary. The Sunday after the youth revival, he tried to talk to his pastor, who put him off and recommended they make an appointment.

"And for some reason that kind of turned me off. I wanted to talk to him right then, so I never made an appointment and he never, that I recall, never came to me to say, 'Larry, we need to talk about that decision.' Well, I just kind of put it on the back burner and joined the military in November 1969."

Looking back, Larry believes he missed God's perfect will by not pursuing missions at that time. The perceived slight by the pastor kindled a spiritual disillusionment that would later grow into a fire of rebellion.

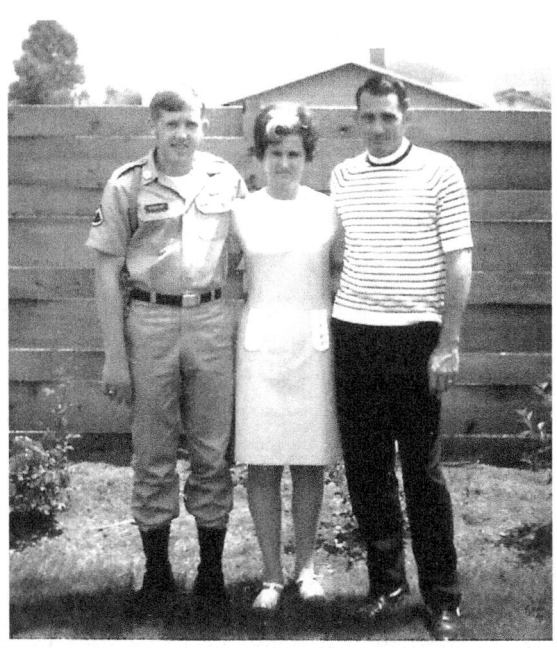

Last goodbyes before leaving for Vietnam. June 1970

ॐ

3
VIETNAM

I enter Larry's bedroom, holding a small glass of milk and a one-ounce pill cup filled with a dozen medications. His eyes are open this morning. He glances in my direction.

"Good morning, Larry." I set the milk and pills on the nightstand.

"Morning, Tom."

The bed creaks. He shuts his eyes and holds his breath. The covers over him shift. His legs and body tense up for several seconds, then relax. I don't think much of it. Sometimes Larry's muscles tighten involuntarily.

"Sleep okay?" I ask and press the incline button on the bed control. Larry's upper body rises to a forty degree angle.

"I've been awake for awhile," he says. "Could you wipe my eyes?"

"Uh huh." I dab the sleep from his closed lids with a tissue. Then I grab the small container of pills. "Ready for some meds?"

"Sip of milk first," he says.

I raise the straw to his lips. He draws in a small amount and sloshes it around in his mouth.

"Here you go," I say and move the pill container toward his lips.

He opens his mouth and I dump all twelve meds in—all at once—and place the straw to his lips. He drinks and gulps, drinks and gulps until all twelve pills are swallowed. Larry is an expert at taking medications.

I attach the blood pressure cuff around his right arm. The cuff inflates.

His legs and body tighten again.

"Are you in pain?" I ask.

"It's been off and on. Kind of a heat sensation."

"How bad is it?" I ask.

He matter-of-factly tells me it's like a red hot poker being rammed up his legs and into his back.

I blink a few times. Yes, I heard him correctly, but my mind can't grasp it.

His blood pressure is higher than normal this morning. I remove the cuff.

Larry's been experiencing neurogenic pain for the last few days and nights. It is caused by faulty signals from the nerves within the damaged myelin sheaths. A recent change in medication dosages hasn't worked out so well and he's waiting for the Veterans Affairs doctor to get back to him with another adjustment. Then the fire will become less frequent and less intense—we hope.

ଐଓଓଃ

When Larry received his high school diploma in June of 1968, the country was reeling over the assassination of presidential candidate Bobby Kennedy just a few days before. Two months earlier, Martin Luther King, Jr. had also succumbed to an assassin's bullet. Riots and protests over the Vietnam War were routine on college campuses throughout the nation.

With short hair and horn-rimmed glasses, Larry, eighteen, looked like a throwback to the innocent days of Ozzie and Harriet. He had yet to fall under the spell of the hippie culture of the sixties, now at its zenith. His main concern upon graduation was finding employment.

He worked a mill job that summer at Weyerhaeuser Lumber Company, and in the fall, attended Lane Community College in Eugene. He lacked motivation, dropped several classes throughout the school year and decided academics weren't for him.

"I just wasn't ready for college," he says, "and so at the end of spring term I went back to work for Weyerhaeuser."

So when 1960's pop guru, Dr. Timothy Leary, advised young people to "turn on, tune in, drop out," Larry did the latter. Although he'd recently begun to smoke cigarettes and drink a few beers, he had yet to turn on to pot or harder drugs. Many years later, Larry would tune in to the living God, though not the false "divinity within" that Leary had in mind.

At nineteen, he rented an apartment with two good friends from high school, Craig Matsler and Steve Keller. Another close friend, a cutup named Tim Ownbey, often hung out with them.

One day, a life insurance salesman came by the apartment and the four buddies listened to his spiel. The salesman told them erroneously that one in four U.S. soldiers serving in the Vietnam War had been killed. The four young men took the salesman at his word and eyed each other in silence.

The actual death rate may have been nearly two percent of those Americans who served (including non-combat military personnel) during the Vietnam War. Of those in the U.S. armed forces who saw actual combat, the death rate may have been between four and six percent. According to National Archive statistics, a total of 58,193 U.S. service men and women died out of 3,403,000 who served in Southeast Asia during the Vietnam War era.

Any chills brought on by the insurance salesman's statistic soon wore off. At the end of the summer of '69, Craig Matsler announced that he and Tim Ownbey had joined the Army. This got Steve Keller and Larry thinking about joining as well. As college students, they'd enjoyed exemption from the draft.

"We [Steve and Larry] weren't going back to school," says Larry, "and we figured that we were probably going to be drafted. So, we went and talked to the Army recruiter and told him that we wanted to go in for two years. And he said, 'Well, you gotta sign up for at least three.' And we said, 'We'll just wait and get drafted then.' Later that day we got a call from the recruiter. He said, 'I think I can work out a deal with you guys.' So he signed us up for two years."

Larry and Steve signed up on the buddy system and

expected to stay together through both basic training and advanced infantry training (AIT). On November 3, 1969, they boarded a bus loaded with several other recruits and traveled to Fort Lewis, Washington for basic training.

"They got us off the bus and had us get into a formation. The first thing the drill sergeant said is, 'I want you to police the area.' Of course, none of us knew what he meant. He had to explain himself. What he wanted us to do was go around and pick up all the paper and cigarette butts off the ground. It's ten o'clock at night, it's cold, it's rainy. And we're thinking to ourselves, 'Boy, did we make a mistake.'"

At one o'clock in the morning, the tired recruits were herded into barracks where they slept, only to be awakened at five o'clock. "The first thing they do is take us down and shave all our heads. My ears were kind of sticking out, so that didn't help matters—I had scars on my head that I hadn't remembered. We all laughed at each other. Then we finally went to breakfast."

For eight weeks, Larry and his cohorts weathered the customary screams and humiliation from drill sergeants. Steve Keller transferred to Fort Hood, Texas for medic training. So much for the buddy system.

Larry continued in AIT for another eight weeks. He and a pal, Gary Benner, signed up for airborne training, hoping to delay going to Vietnam. A week later Larry's company received orders to go to Panama to guard the canal, thus avoiding Vietnam. But Larry and Gary missed out. They flew to Fort Benning, Georgia for four weeks of airborne training.

"The first three weeks was training and drilling on how to jump out of a plane and how to land correctly—a lot of exercise, a lot of running, a lot of physical training. I was probably in the best shape of my life when I came out of airborne."

Larry and Gary then signed up for rigger slinging school. Rigger slingers packed parachutes destined for drop loads. "It seemed like a good idea because that way you weren't out in the field, fighting."

At that time they also signed up for pathfinder school, which meant they could stay in the States for another four weeks. In the Vietnam War, pathfinders determined the best helicopter landing sites and withdrawal routes in war zones. They performed ground-level air traffic control as well.

A mix-up occurred since they'd also signed up for rigger slinging school. Ultimately, the Army decided to train Larry and Gary as pathfinders. Four weeks later, they graduated.

"And sure enough we got orders to Vietnam."

The men were given a thirty day leave. Larry flew home to visit family and friends before heading to Southeast Asia.

Early in the morning on June 19, 1970, Larry boarded a plane at the deportation center in Oakland, California. "It was a 22-hour flight to Vietnam," he says. "We flew to Hawaii, then to Wake Island, and then the Philippines. It was about a seven hour flight from the Philippines to Vietnam. And at that point everybody really began thinking about where they were going. Most of the flight from the Philippines to Vietnam was fairly quiet, not a lot of talking. So we arrived in Vietnam in late evening at Bien Hoa airbase. We got off the plane and they loaded us up in buses."

The busload of recruits traveled through the city of Bien Hoa to a nearby location in South Vietnam where they obtained their orders. Larry expected to receive his pathfinder assignment. Instead, he was assigned to the 1st Battalion 12th Cavalry D Company 3rd Platoon.

He'd been assigned to the infantry, not pathfinders.

"I told the guy, 'Wait a minute. I'm a pathfinder.' And he

said, 'Well, I don't know what to tell you, but that's where you're going.'"

So due to another mix-up, Larry became an infantry foot soldier. His odds for survival would be considerably less than a pathfinder's.

His company spent a week learning about the country and what to watch out for. Then they boarded helicopters and flew to their base of operation, or firebase, called LZ (landing zone) Buttons.

"Our company was out in the field and so they just dropped us off," he recalls. "Nobody would tell us anything. It was monsoon season and it was raining pretty hard, so we tried to put together a hooch or a tent. Well, about midnight the thing caved in. So here we were all soaked and looking for a dry place to sleep. I found a big tent that had all the supplies in it. So I went in there and just slept on the floor."

From LZ Buttons, soldiers were flown by helicopter, or CAA'd (combat air assault), to various locations where they would embark on search-and-destroy missions lasting up to twenty-three days each.

"The missions were usually to find something of the enemy's and destroy it. Or if we were told they were operating in that vicinity, we were to try and find them and capture them or kill them."

Larry felt no qualms about this lethal objective. After all, the enemy had killed thousands of American soldiers—and they were trying to kill him.

At night, the troops prepared for mortar attacks by digging foxholes big enough to hold two men. They used their ponchos as tents to sleep in and ate rations stored in their backpacks. "I wasn't really afraid," says Larry. "I guess the only thing I really thought about was, '*Am I going to live through it?*'"

The first mission took place in wet, mountainous terrain. Larry's platoon spent much of the time struggling up slippery slopes. "It would be so slick going up the mountain that you'd take two or three steps and slide back five or six."

The enemy failed to appear. After four or five days of miserable rain and drudgery, a helicopter picked them up and they returned to LZ Buttons for a day.

Larry became friends with a Cambodian soldier called Ace, who had earned the nickname due to his many skills. Adept at observation and infiltrating NVA troops, Ace had once killed a North Vietnamese general. A bounty was placed on his head.

He and Larry were in the same platoon. "We'd sit down and have a cigarette together," says Larry. "He talked English pretty good and told me stories. He'd been fighting since he was a young boy."

Ace was somebody you wanted by your side in a firefight.

The second mission began at night. Helicopters dropped the troops off near the Cambodian border. They entered a major trail known to be well-traveled by NVA (North Vietnamese Army) and Vietcong (South Vietnamese communist guerillas allied with the NVA). Larry's company walked in darkness five or six hundred yards and pitched camp.

At each end of the camp, they set up automatic ambushes, consisting of tripwires connected to Claymore mines. Each mine contained 750 bb-sized pellets. If an enemy soldier stumbled over the tripwire, the mine would explode. Says Larry, "It would let us know that the enemy was in the area and it would kill a few of them."

At about six in the morning Larry awoke with the rest of the company. He drank some hot chocolate and chatted for a half hour with a young soldier named Clarence, a newlywed from

Pennsylvania. His wife was expecting a child.

Boom! A Claymore mine exploded. Seconds passed. A gunshot fired. Silence.

A small patrol from Larry's company went out to investigate. They found two NVA soldiers, dead, at the edge of the camp. The patrol speculated that one of the victims committed suicide because he was still alive after his legs were blown off. This explained the gunshot.

A warrior by nature, Larry felt little fear and saw the enemy deaths as a good thing. "And so we knew that these were probably scouts and they were in the area. Our captain had radioed back to headquarters and asked the colonel if we could break brush instead of following the trail, because we figured that they might be up ahead waiting to ambush us."

The colonel said no, ordering the company to stay on the trail. This insured they'd engage the enemy. But it placed the Americans at a significant disadvantage, greatly increasing their visibility. They'd be sitting ducks for the hidden NVA.

The Americans broke camp and headed up the trail. The company of forty-five men divided into three platoons. The first platoon walked point (in front). The second platoon covered the middle, and the third, Larry's, stayed in back.

They encountered a stream. Crossing would make them vulnerable. They'd be wide open and slow, due to wading. The sergeant ordered Larry and Ace to hustle ahead and pull security in the middle of the stream. So they stood guard in the stream while the entire company crossed and reentered the trail. The pair then waded quickly to catch up.

Still in the stream, Larry and Ace saw movement beyond the bank to the right. An NVA soldier darted near the trail. Larry put his M-16 on automatic and shot at him. Ace did the same. "We really don't know whether or not we shot him because we didn't go out to investigate," says Larry.

They hustled to catch up with the company. Ace ran ahead. Larry slowed in front of a huge fallen tree that blocked the trail.

A bullet whizzed by his head. Then another.

"I hurried across the log and kind of hid underneath it. My sergeant was about thirty or forty yards ahead. He kept waving for me to get up front because the first platoon was under fire where they had run into an ambush."

Larry hesitated. If he moved from the log, he'd be an open target. The sergeant kept yelling. Larry sprang from his cover. He sprinted past the sergeant to the firefight.

"So I raced to the front and saw these friends of mine coming back. One friend had been shot in the arm three times, different locations."

The initial onslaught had passed when Larry caught up with the company. He took cover behind a tree. Scattered gunshots continued—but the NVA soldiers had struck quickly and disappeared.

"They told us if you could live through the first four seconds of a firefight," says Larry, "your chances of survival were good, because it's within that initial blast of the ambush when you're not able to get down to protect yourself that they get you."

The gunfire ceased. Larry surveyed the disaster. He saw a soldier lying still on the ground. Larry asked the harried lieutenant if the fallen soldier was alive. The officer didn't know. Larry knelt down to see.

"I rolled him over and he had a bullet right between the eyes—blew out the back of his head. It happened to be the same guy [Clarence] that I was talking to that morning who had just gotten married in September. He'd come into the company with me—we'd only been there ten days."

This image of Clarence branded itself into Larry's psyche. It came to represent the horror of the Vietnam War.

Forty years later, the sight of Clarence is still sharp and vivid in his mind's eye. Time refuses to dull the memory. Though he knows otherwise, Larry feels as if Clarence died only moments ago.

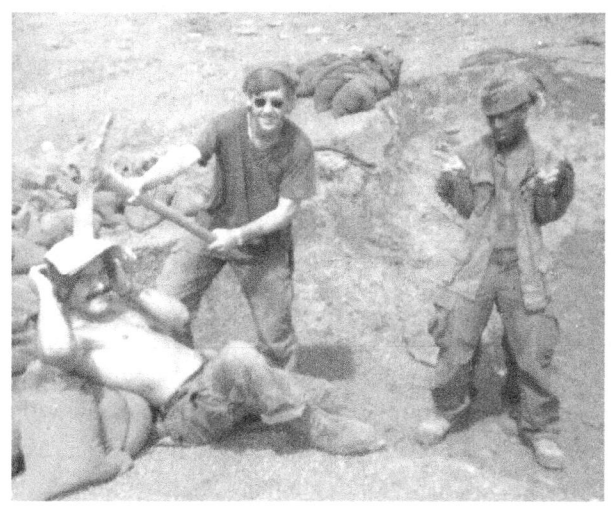

Larry horsing around with his buddies. Vietnam, 1970

༄༅

4

WOUNDED SOUL

I wheel Larry into the living room and park him next to the pellet stove. He enjoys the full blast of warm air. Larry chills easily, largely because he can't move his muscles to build up body heat. The Browning home is too warm for me, but not for the ruler of the house, Miss Kitty, who sleeps serenely in an easy chair in the corner of the living room.

It's the day before Thanksgiving 2009 and Ann busies herself about the home, preparing for tomorrow's big family feast. The turkey still thaws in the basement.

"Could I get some coffee?" asks Larry.

"You bet," I say and head to the nearby kitchen where I fill his customized mug. It has a straw taped to it for easier sipping. I work three of his fingers through the mug's handle so it stays secure in his hand. It takes me a few tries to position his arm just right so the straw is near his lips. He draws in a sip. "Ah."

I clock out for the day, but instead of leaving, pour a cup of joe for myself and scoot a dining chair next to Larry. I fetch my travel bag from the kitchen and pull out a tape recorder. "Ready when you are."

"Okay," says Larry.

I clear my throat and press the record button. We continue to discuss the Vietnam War and its aftermath. Larry explains that, at age twenty, he believed the Vietnam conflict was a just cause. "We were trying to protect South Vietnam from becoming communist, so I thought that was a worthwhile endeavor."

His priorities changed after the ambush. Although he continued to view the war as justifiable, winning it became a secondary goal. "You realized that the most important thing was to protect your buddies. It wasn't so much you were fighting for a cause as you were fighting for your life and the life of your friends."

"How were you received by people when you got home?" I ask.

"I don't think that I told anybody I was a Vietnam veteran because of the feelings [of student protestors], and the riots that took place. That's why we grew our hair long and everything, so we'd kind of fit in with the crowd."

He himself did not experience hostility from protestors. "But I know there were other vets that were called baby-killers."

Not exactly a hero's welcome. I take a sip of coffee and ask Larry when he first experienced post-traumatic stress disorder.

"I would say it was only a few years ago that I actually

admitted to it," he says. "I just kind of kept my feelings to myself. Even today, I still think about, and dream about, events that took place forty years ago in the war. It just seems strange that, after forty years, you still can't shake it. I mean, I dream about those things a lot more than I dream about anything else. And there are times at night when I'll lie awake for a couple hours, at least, thinking about the experiences in Vietnam."

The warm air from the pellet stove hits me in the face and aggravates my already dry, burning eyes. "So, it was recently that you acknowledged having PTSD. Was that also when you were diagnosed with it?"

Larry draws in some coffee through the straw. "Yeah, I was diagnosed with it in 2008. I probably recognized it some time ago, but I tried to repress the fact that I might have it. I was interviewed once before about PTSD, and I told the guy [VA psychiatrist] that I didn't have it because of my faith. So I kind of used that as an out, you know, to say that I didn't believe I should have something like that because I was a Christian."

Larry's statement surprises me—that it took him most of his adult life to admit to having PTSD. I ask if he experienced symptoms in the years just after the war.

Symptoms occurred, but he lived in heavy denial during that period. "It's probably because I stayed stoned for about ten or twelve years—that way I didn't have to deal with it."

Larry and the VA psychiatrist agree that the recent flare-ups of PTSD are due to the countless hours Larry spends sitting and thinking. He's unable to distract himself with physical activity, so he's left with excessively large amounts of time to think about the war.

"What are typical symptoms of PTSD and what are yours?" I ask.

"I think typical symptoms are a constant, where there are

dreams, sometimes nightmares. Every time I hear a helicopter go overhead, it takes me back to Vietnam. I remember when I first got out of the service—if I'd hear a car backfire, I'd hit the ground. So I think a lot of the PTSD is just the recurring dreams you can't shake. I know the psychiatrist that I talked to called them nightmares, which in some ways they are, because you relive them time and time again. What happened wasn't a very pretty picture, you know."

ଚ୦ଔ

Larry's first encounter with the enemy saw four men dead and eight wounded. Within minutes of the ambush, U.S. Cobra gunships and Huey helicopters flew overhead, searching for the North Vietnamese troops. Medevac choppers arrived and picked up the wounded, but not the dead. Reports came in that the North Vietnamese company responsible for the ambush had been located. Larry never heard whether they received retribution.

The rest of the day elapsed like a confusing blur to Larry. Nightfall arrived and the fallen soldiers still hadn't been airlifted out. The company camped in a perimeter, or circle, around the bodies. This enabled them to guard every side, similar to what the old wagon trains did at the end of a travel day.

After a day of loud chaos, a silent gloom settled over the encampment. The soldiers could see the gray-green body bags in the moonlight.

Unable to sleep, Larry sat against a tree most of the night and stared at the dead lying in the perimeter's center. The twenty-year-old tried to make sense of the tragedy, tried to grasp the big picture, the purpose of the war.

As the hours passed, clarity emerged. Larry experienced an epiphany.

"I got to thinking—here we were shooting at people we didn't know, who we had no personal grudge against. And they were doing the same. It was at that point I realized it wasn't so much that we were fighting for South Vietnam's freedom, but it became more personal—we were fighting for each other's lives, and the whole purpose was to stay alive."

He had heard it before, the critical need to watch your fellow soldiers' backs. The words had been emphasized and certainly taken seriously. But now Larry's foremost aim became to protect his fellow soldiers and himself.

He intended to do whatever it took to accomplish this newfound purpose.

Early the next morning, a medevac chopper flew in and removed the four bodies. Having also lost eight to injuries, the company numbered only thirty-three soldiers, down from the original forty-five. They broke camp and continued up the jungle trail. Around midmorning they stopped to rest near a small clearing.

The company received news that the battalion colonel would fly in soon for a visit. A sergeant paired Larry with another soldier and assigned them to OP (observation post) in the jungle across the clearing from the company. A second pair of guards was assigned to a different location. Larry and his partner hid in dense brush about seventy yards away from their company and watched for enemy movement.

The colonel's Huey flew in and landed near where the three platoons rested. Larry and the other guard observed this from the other side of the clearing.

The company's captain walked toward the chopper. The colonel stepped out and greeted the saluting captain.

The sight of the colonel ignited a silent rage within Larry. All the chaos, anguish and death of the previous day coalesced into pure hatred toward this one man.

The day before, the captain had radioed the colonel with a request for the company to stay off the trail and break brush. This would have kept the Americans hidden and given them a better chance at seeing the enemy first. Due to the earlier deaths of the two NVA scouts from the claymore mine explosions, the North Vietnamese became aware of the Americans' location. Sticking to the trail invited the ambush. The colonel denied the captain's request and ordered the company to stay on the trail to insure they would engage the enemy.

Larry believed this decision resulted in the ambush. The colonel had a reputation for putting men at unnecessary risk.

"All of us in the company believed he was responsible for the deaths of the [four] men," says Larry. "He was disdained by every soldier that ever served under him."

Larry wanted nothing less than to kill him. Though vengeful anger provided the primary motivation, he also had a logical justification. By eliminating the colonel, Larry rationalized he would protect the lives of the soldiers within his own company as well as future soldiers serving under the colonel's command.

Larry expressed these sentiments to the other guard, who nodded in agreement. They arrived at a decision.

The colonel must die.

And because the two sentries were hidden in dense jungle brush, they could probably pull off the assassination without being spotted.

While the colonel and captain talked near the idling Huey, the two guards hatched a rapid-fire plan. Larry had earned an expert ranking—the highest—with an M16. He would shoot the colonel while the other guard fired into the jungle, as a ruse, at nonexistent enemy soldiers. This way, NVA snipers would receive blame for the colonel's death. Though the plan contained flaws, a better opportunity seemed unlikely.

"He [the colonel] seemed kind of jovial with our captain, and that just added to my anger," says Larry.

Hidden in the jungle, about seventy yards away from the target, Larry and his co-conspirator positioned themselves.

Larry raised his M16. He aimed it at the helmeted colonel's chest.

"The thing about the M16," says Larry, "is that whenever it hits a person, the bullet tumbles. It can go in at your shoulder and come out at your knee. So it does a lot of damage when it hits a person."

Larry's right thumb touched the safety. Anger continued to burn, along with a hint of nervousness. His forefinger inched toward the trigger. He inhaled deeply.

Rational thoughts surfaced: *he could end up in military prison or be shot by a firing squad. This would be murder, the ultimate violation of the faith of his youth.* These twin realizations of consequence and conscience combined to overcome his anger.

Larry lowered the weapon.

No gushing sense of relief occurred. He still wanted the colonel dead. "I was hoping that we could get ambushed again and the enemy would take care of it for us, you know, because we certainly wouldn't try to stop him from being shot."

The oblivious commander concluded his meeting with the captain and boarded the helicopter. Barely ten minutes had passed from the Huey's landing until it took off. Within that short time Larry nearly succumbed to ultimate folly, but opted for wisdom. He would make plenty of bad choices during the next decade, but none that matched the calamitous result had he pulled the trigger that day.

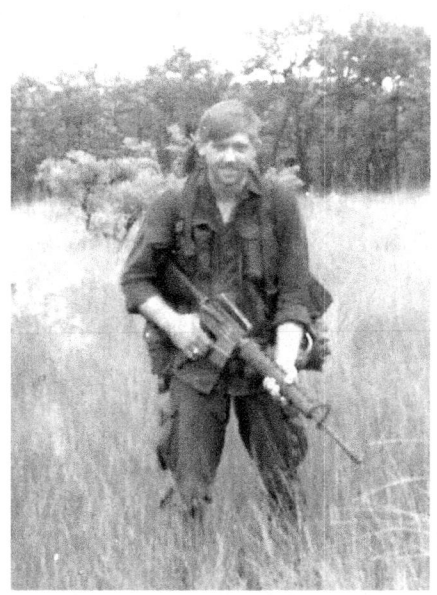

"Me again with my trusty M-16."
Vietnam, 1970

☙◌ℭ

5

ONE IN FOUR DIE

I drive the wheelchair van into the parking lot of the
Eugene Veterans' Affairs clinic. Spaces are scarce.

"Park in the back," says Larry, seated in the passenger
side, his wheelchair safely locked to the floor.

"Okey-dokey," I say and maneuver around the building.
Sure enough, there's plenty of parking on the back side. I pull
into a handicapped spot near the entrance.

Still unaccustomed to the various buttons and controls

specific to the wheelchair van, I hesitate a few seconds while searching the dash for the floor-lock release button.

"Unbuckle me first," says Larry.

"Oh, yeah," I say. "Getting ahead of myself again." My job duties are very sequential—first things first, one thing after the other. It challenges my zigzagging, nonlinear mind. I unbuckle Larry and notice two identical buttons on the left side of the dash. One releases the floor lock. "Let's see, is it the left or right button?" I'm afraid if I press the wrong one, something might explode.

"Left," says Larry, going by memory. "Be ready to back the wheelchair out as soon as you push it or it'll relock."

"Okay," I say and reach over Larry's shoulder to turn on the power to the wheelchair. That's right. I also have to deal with the electric wheelchair controls. During the last year, Larry lost the use of his right hand, so he can no longer operate the wheelchair. My right hand is on the chair's steering toggle, which doubles as a forward and reverse throttle; my left forefinger is ready to push the van's floor-lock release button. I push and hear the click of the lock releasing. My right hand pulls the wheelchair toggle in reverse. The wheelchair jerks backward and stops abruptly. Larry's head lurches forward, then back. He raises an eyebrow. I hear the floor lock re-latch. Fortunately, the wheelchair is free—with Larry still in it.

Larry gives me a side-glance. "You're getting better," he says.

"Uh, thanks," I say, relieved that he still has a sense of humor—and no whiplash. Good thing there's a VA clinic nearby.

A video game aficionado could easily operate the less-than-responsive wheelchair toggle. I'm bad at video games. More technical challenges ensue as I struggle through the process of getting Larry safely down the wheelchair ramp and onto pavement. We exit the van unscathed.

"Enter through the front," says my patient boss.

I weave the wheelchair along a narrow cement walkway past the left side of the building until we arrive at the front. The VA has an automatic, motion-activated door that slides open. That's nice, because it's a hassle pushing a wheelchair through doors that want to spring closed.

We enter the building, move through the foyer and turn left toward the check-in counter. There's not much of a line and soon the receptionist takes Larry's appointment card. She fiddles with a computer, smiles and directs us to the main waiting area.

Now we experience the "hurry up and wait" syndrome. About a half dozen men sit in chairs, waiting to see a doctor or nurse practitioner. Most appear to be in their late fifties or sixties. Two are old enough to be Korean War vets. Larry is the only one in a wheelchair. Several minutes pass and a nurse calls Larry into an exam room, where she checks his vitals. The doctor arrives and asks Larry some questions.

We go to another sitting area to await a blood draw. Those in the room keep to themselves. I hear a loud voice down a hallway. A tall, strong-looking man in his early fifties, with shoulder-length hair, talks forcefully into his cell phone as he walks toward the waiting area. He complains about his treatment by the VA and how they've failed to adequately treat his kidney problem. He describes how he's informed various news media about his plight; I deduce that he's currently talking to a representative from a local television station. This goes on for a few minutes while the rest of us sit and try to appear as if we're not eavesdropping. The man eventually leaves.

I turn to my boss and state the obvious. "Sounds like he's not happy with the VA."

Larry nods and says, "The VA's been good to me."

છ⁂ભ

The colonel, clueless that he'd nearly been shot, ended his conversation with the captain. He boarded the chopper, which lifted off and flew away.

Private Browning wished him the worst.

Larry's battered company pulled on their packs and resumed the mission. They stayed on the trail for the next four or five days. An NVA battalion had been spotted about a mile away, moving toward the Americans. The reduced company was critically outnumbered and had to leave or risk being slaughtered.

"At that time," says Larry, "because we had eight guys wounded and four killed—we were down to thirty-three men. We were waiting for the helicopters to come and pick us up. That morning they finally arrived. By the time they got us, the NVA battalion was only a half mile away from us, so we got out of there just in the nick of time."

The company returned to the fire base, LZ Buttons, for some rest. "We would go out for [as many as] twenty-three days at a time and then come back in and stay at the fire base for seven days. We'd pull security on the fire base and it also was a time to relax."

Rock music from Armed Forces Radio often played at the base. Larry and his buddies would climb on top of the bunkers and sing along to the war protest classic, *I Feel Like I'm Fixin' to Die*.

This didn't mean they opposed the Vietnam conflict. Larry and his pals wanted very much to crush the communists in the north. Although they supported the premise of stopping communism, they still had doubts about the war.

Many of Larry's fellow soldiers believed that the U.S. government wasn't giving the war a full effort. It became increasingly clear that the political leaders wanted out of the conflict more than they wanted to win it. A halfhearted war effort seemed futile to the troops.

And the corruption that plagued South Vietnam's government and military leadership had a demoralizing effect on soldiers.

Why was Larry fighting? The answer was murky. One thing was clear, though—he'd fight to keep himself and his buddies alive.

The horrors of combat typically come to mind when people talk about war. And fighting is indeed the worst part. But oftentimes unmentioned are the numerous physical hardships faced by soldiers apart from combat. The swarms of mosquitoes in Vietnam were a continual nuisance and health risk. During one search-and-destroy mission, Larry's platoon spent a week at the top of a ridge so thick with mosquitoes that if you opened your mouth, bunches would fly in. "You were constantly trying to bat them from your face. You'd smoke to keep the mosquitoes away."

Larry awoke one morning to find his backpack infested with termites. He spent several minutes cleaning it out. After breakfast, he put on his helmet and got ready to go. Something scurried in his hair and scalp. "So I took my helmet off and...the whole inside was full of termites. And they were crawling all over my hair and down my neck. It took me awhile to get rid of them."

The third mission posed a particularly tough physical challenge. Combat air assault helicopters dropped the company off into a field of elephant grass, which reached ten to fifteen feet high. The choppers couldn't land, so the men jumped out. The soldiers found themselves in nearly three feet of water. "They hadn't told us, but the field was completely surrounded by a river."

They spent two weeks in knee- to waist-high water. At the end of each day they'd look for tiny islands large enough for at least one man. "So here you sat all night with your feet almost in the water and raining all night. It was pretty miserable."

At the end of two weeks they encountered soggy marshland. Dry legs were nice, except for one thing—the wet ground was infested with leaches. "Every time we'd take a step, we'd look down, and there were these little inch-long leeches that were trying to get up your pant legs to get on you. They were falling out of the trees, I mean they were everywhere. There were thousands of them. We finally got to the river and we actually had to call in a helicopter to drop out a bunch of bug spray so we could kill all the leeches."

The wet, soggy, miserable mission lasted twenty-three days. Because of the constant moisture, Larry contracted a painful skin ailment. The hair follicles on his legs, from the knees down, became inflamed with painful boils. He could barely lace up his boots because of the swelling. Larry requested time off to heal, but the major denied the request and sent Larry on another mission. After three or four days in the jungle, his legs turned red and blue. Liquid oozed from the boils. He could no longer lace his boots.

"Finally I told my sergeant to hold up, and the captain came back and he said, 'What's going on?' I said, 'Either you guys get me out of here, or medevac me out of here, and get me to a doctor that can look at these legs. Or you can just leave me here because I can't go any further.'"

Larry got his wish. A medevac chopper picked him up from the field and took him to a simple aid station in Phuc Vinh for treatment. They soaked his legs in a Betadine solution and assigned him to guard duty two hours a night at a far outpost called the green line. Mosquitoes attacked him badly there.

This lasted for two or three days and his legs failed to improve. "So they sent me to the 15th Med, which was a hospital kind of like the MASH unit you saw on TV." They prescribed penicillin and stopped giving him quinine, which he'd taken daily for malaria prevention.

Larry stayed at the 15th Med a little over a week. One night, the North Vietnamese launched mortars at the hospital. Patients were quickly moved to bunkers. Fortunately, there were no casualties.

Larry's legs remained infected, so he caught a chopper to a larger hospital, 24th Evac, in the city of Long Binh. A dermatologist performed a biopsy and diagnosed it as folliculitis, a curable infection.

A few days after the biopsy, Larry suffered splitting headaches, cold sweats and a high temperature. A blood sample revealed he had falciparum malaria, the most deadly form of the disease. He had most likely caught it from the mosquitoes that attacked him a week or so earlier while on guard duty in Phuc Vinh. The upside? Most victims survive, and once it's cured it doesn't recur like other forms of malaria.

A one-star general visited Larry one morning at the hospital and asked why he'd caught malaria. Larry said he'd been taken off quinine. The general seemed concerned, so Larry figured somebody would face some type of reprimand for withdrawing the quinine.

Penicillin hadn't cured the folliculitis, so they ordered a different antibiotic. "Finally it started getting better," he says. "I spent about two weeks at 24th Evac, where my legs cleared up. But because I had malaria, they sent me to the 22nd Convalescent Center along the South China Sea. It was a convalescent-type home where people who were recovering from wounds or malaria had time to regain their strength. I spent about two weeks there."

His doctor happened to be a fellow Oregonian. He assigned Larry to light duty with plenty of free time. The convalescent center had an outdoor theater by the sea, complete with bleachers and a big screen. One night, as Larry and other patients watched a movie, the Vietcong or NVA, in boats just off the coast, attacked the Americans with machine guns. No one was hurt, but it made for quite a show.

One morning during Larry's stay at the convalescent center, the body of an American soldier was discovered on the beach. He'd overdosed on heroin, the needle still in his arm. "Well," says Larry, "a lot of the heroin that came into Vietnam came through the South China Sea. And it was almost pure, so those guys that had used heroin in the United States were used to a diluted form. Because of that, there were numerous cases of guys overdosing."

During the Vietnam War, soldiers had easy access to inexpensive marijuana, opium and heroin. Larry remembers a Jeep ride he took with two medics. They stopped at the side of the road and one of the medics ran into a shack. "He came back and I asked them what they were doing. They told me they were buying some drugs, buying some heroin. I said, 'That's enough. I don't need to know any more.'"

After nearly forty days of treatment at the various medical facilities, Larry finally recovered from the folliculitis and malaria. Vacation over, he rejoined his company.

After a month back in the field, Larry's company took a three or four day break or "stand-down" in Bien Hoa, the location of the division headquarters. While there, the soldiers were told to check their records to see if they'd received any awards or medals. Larry's records weren't there, so he asked where they were.

"And the guy that was working down there told me,

'Well, you've been transferred.' I said, 'Transferred? Transferred to where?' He said, 'You've been transferred to headquarters 11th Aviation Group 3rd Pathfinder Team.' And I said, 'When was I supposed to report?' He said, 'You were supposed to report a month ago.'"

Larry took a copy of the orders to the first sergeant's office and demanded to know why he wasn't told about the transfer. The sergeant claimed ignorance about the order. Larry noticed a copy of his transfer near the desk, evidence that the sergeant knew. The short-handed infantry needed to retain as many soldiers as possible. "Yeah," said the sergeant, "you've been transferred, so you need to turn in your gear and take your orders and go to the military base and get a flight to Phuc Vinh."

So Larry would finally become a pathfinder, the position he should have been assigned at the very start of his tour. Again, pathfinders were much more likely to survive war than infantry soldiers. Larry's previous four months of high-risk foot-soldiering had been the unnecessary result of mixed-up paperwork.

He wrote a goodbye note to his buddies in the company and paid for two cases of beer to be delivered to them. Then he caught a flight to Phuc Vinh and arrived at the 3rd Pathfinder team headquarters.

"I walked in and the captain was sitting at his desk. I threw my orders down and he says, 'We were wondering where you were at.' And it was kind of like they hadn't been too upset that I wasn't there, you know. I could have probably just traveled around Vietnam till my tour was up and nobody would have ever missed me."

After two leisurely weeks at the pathfinders headquarters, Larry caught a one-hour chopper flight to an Air Force battalion airstrip "in the middle of nowhere" called Fire Support Base Mace. He spent a week there directing air traffic in and out.

He was then assigned (about one hundred miles from Mace) to an engineering compound near a village called Phu Lam. Aircraft and gun ships refueled and rearmed at the compound. Larry lived and worked there for the next two months. He and another pathfinder directed air traffic in and out of the compound from six in the morning until six at night. Only one pathfinder needed to be on duty during any one shift, which resulted in plenty of time off.

Larry smoked pot for the first time while there. But he felt the drug clouded his mind enough to hinder his work. So he didn't smoke it again until after Vietnam.

"It was pretty easy duty. It was a lot better than pounding the brush. Every night I had a bed that I could get into that was nice and comfortable."

One day, Larry spotted an Army Times newspaper inside the large tent barracks at the compound. He skimmed through the news and read the obituaries of all the soldiers who had died the previous week. His heart sank at the sight of a familiar name. Tim Ownbey, Larry's close friend from Springfield, was listed among the casualties. He and two other soldiers had died on October 25 when a Claymore mine exploded.

Eugene's *The Register-Guard* columnist, Bob Welch, in a 1996 feature article commemorating Ownbey, quoted from a letter by Wesley Sisco, who served in Tim's company: "We had set out an automatic ambush, a type of booby trap, several days before. We came back to check it out and remove it. But 'Charlie' had found the trap and reversed it right by our battery. When they picked it up, they tripped the ambush. It got all three men instantly."

Larry would learn the details of Tim's death later. "We had become very close friends," says Larry, "so I was really upset to hear that Tim had been killed."

On Christmas Eve, about two months after Tim Ownbey's death, Larry was temporarily monitoring a radio and received a message:

"Is Larry Browning there?"

"Yeah, this is him."

"Larry, you need to get on a helicopter and head back to Mace as soon as possible."

"What's going on?" asked Larry.

"Well, you just need to get on a helicopter and come back."

Later that day, he caught a chopper heading to fire base Mace. There, a lieutenant asked him, "Do you have any dress greens?"

Totally in the dark about what was going on, Larry said, "No." He wondered where the officer expected him to get dress greens.

The lieutenant explained nothing, only telling Larry to immediately fly to the headquarters in Phuc Vinh.

He caught the next chopper to Phuc Vinh. There, the captain and the first sergeant ushered him into a back room.

One of them said, "We don't know how to tell you this, but we just got news that your father was killed in a logging accident. You need to get home right away."

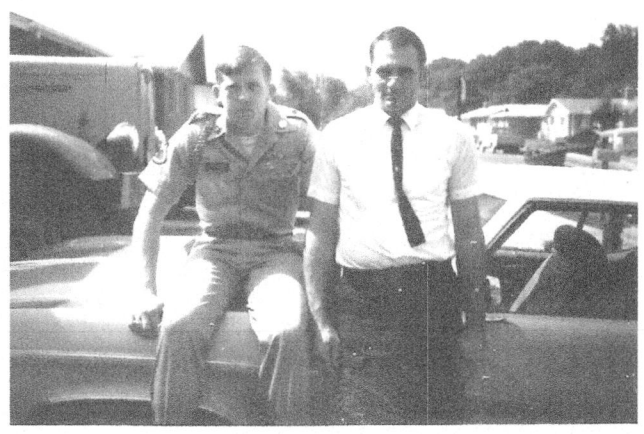

Larry with his father, just before the flight to Vietnam. June, 1970

ဆာ

6

HOME FOR CHRISTMAS

Larry's mother, Agatha Morse, sits across from me in a recliner in the Browning living room. Her sixty-year-old son sits next to her in his wheelchair. The pellet stove blasts him with warm air. Outside, sunshine and blue skies belie warmth on this cool September afternoon, the last day of summer, 2010.

Agatha is here for her weekly visit with Larry, and she's graciously allowed me to interview her. I ask about her childhood in North Carolina and discover she was born in the Appalachian Mountains on October 25, 1929, four days before the stock market crashed.

"I caused it," she quips.

Growing up during the Great Depression, Agatha remembers her father scrambling for any work he could find. "We didn't have a car. It was probably over a mile that we would walk and go to church."

Agatha first met Jay Browning in childhood. She played house with his sisters and managed to convince Jay, four years her senior, to join the fun and pretend to be her husband. Not that she had any ideas. True romance kindled several years later, when Jay returned from his World War II service in the Navy. They married on November 14, 1947.

She describes Jay as a zealous Christian who frequently shared his faith. He worked hard as a church deacon and regularly gave up his Saturdays to work on church construction projects.

"He said 'Amen!' a lot in services," says Agatha. "He was about the only one who would say, 'Amen.' And a lot of times, when they'd pray at church, Jay would get down on his knees in front of the pew. No matter who was praying, Jay kneeled. There weren't many people down there who were doing that then."

Agatha recounts the day she heard the news of her husband's death on December 22, 1970. She was driving home from her job as a nurse at Eugene's Sacred Heart Hospital and expected to see Jay. They planned to take their daughter Brenda and her husband Dennis out for their wedding anniversary. As Agatha approached home, she saw the family doctor and a couple from her church standing in the driveway.

"I knew something had happened and I stopped the car right in the middle of the street, got out and said, 'What's wrong?'"

The doctor said, "Jay was killed this afternoon."

"I could not believe it," she recalls. "I just started screaming. I told whoever was there to go get Brenda. Then he [the doctor] tried to tell me what he had heard—something happened to the log truck and it rolled over Jay."

Agatha tells how she and Jay had prayed that Larry would be allowed to come home for Christmas. They'd even purchased an airline ticket and mailed it to Larry's headquarters. The ticket was useless. The Army notified them that the quota had already been filled for soldiers coming home.

"That just shows when you pray," says Agatha, "you never know how God's going to answer. Larry got home on Christmas Day."

I ask how she dealt with grief in the period after Jay's death. She mentions that her nursing job provided a good distraction, keeping her away from the house during the day.

She tears up. "After he'd been gone about seven months, I thought I was going to lose my mind. I just thought, *He's gone and he's not coming back."*

"Who supported you during this time?" I ask.

Without hesitation, she says, "My church."

Needless to say, they didn't celebrate Brenda's anniversary that night. "She [Brenda] was devastated, just like I was," says Agatha. "She and Larry were really close to Jay. Jay was a jolly person. He loved to have fun and they'd dance around the house when there was music on. They were just really close"

∞∞

Larry stared in disbelief at the captain and first sergeant. On Christmas Eve, 1970, in a back room of Army headquarters in Phuc Vinh, South Vietnam, Larry tried to process the news of his father's death. The sheer distance—Springfield, Oregon being nearly halfway around the world—made it seem all the more unreal. Within moments, though, reality sunk in.

"I broke down," says Larry, "because my dad and I were really close. I broke down and cried."

The final conversation between father and son had occurred over the phone three months earlier while Larry recovered from malaria at the convalescent center by the South China Sea. Agatha had shared the line with Jay. "He was his jovial self," says Larry. "He was very outgoing. He was kind of a character."

Within hours of hearing the news of his father's death, Larry caught a helicopter to Bien Hoa Airbase. He was granted a thirty-day leave. That night he called home and talked to his mother and sister. They confirmed Jay's death, which occurred December 22nd.

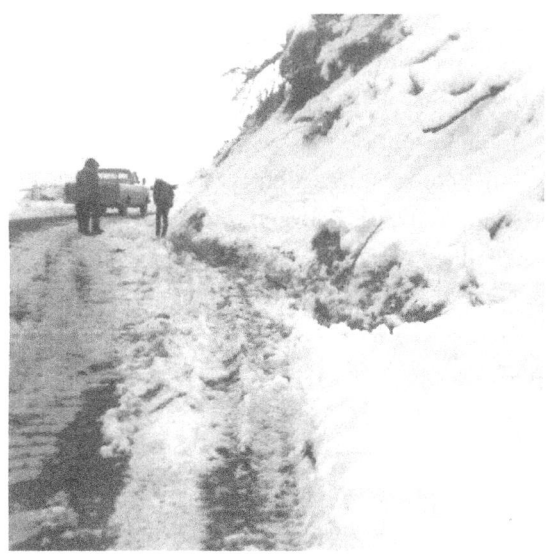

The site of Jay's passing, a few days after the accident

On Christmas morning, 1970, Larry boarded a commercial airliner out of Bien Hoa. After a stopover in Oakland, he caught a flight to Eugene, Oregon. An uncle drove him to Springfield. Because of the time change, it was still Christmas morning when he arrived home. In essence, he experienced two Christmases, awful as they were. A nice gift emerged, however. Unknown to Larry, he had left Vietnam for good.

He showed up at his family home still dressed in jungle fatigues. His mom, sister, aunt and grandmother greeted him.

"And you know," he says, "it was a very sobering time. I wanted to go to the funeral home and see Dad, so I went down with my uncle and spent a little time alone with Dad."

The next day Larry visited the logging site in the hills where his father died. Jay had operated a self-loading log truck. The day of the accident, someone saw him at the landing site, checking the binders that secure logs to the truck. The ground had been icy and slick that day.

No one saw the accident, but as Jay drove down the hill, the truck probably slid out of control. He may have figured the truck was moving toward a cliff-like embankment so he engaged the Jake brake. The truck kept sliding, so he likely jumped out to avoid tumbling down the embankment. The back dual wheels ran over him and crushed his midsection.

A man found Jay still alive moments after he'd been crushed. Jay's last words were, "I've been run over by my truck. Go and get help."

Minutes later, Jay, age forty-four, was dead.

Two or three days after the funeral, Larry had a dream about his father. "In the dream we met one morning and sat and talked. We walked together, spent the whole day together, just doing different things. And at the end of the day, Dad said, 'Well, you know I gotta go.' And I said, 'Yeah, I know, Dad.' And I started weeping. So I hugged Dad goodbye and he kind of walked away. I woke up and tears were just streaming down my face. I really felt that the Lord had given me an opportunity that I had really longed for, just to spend the day with my dad. Whether it was just a dream or a vision, it was so real."

During the thirty day leave, Larry spent a good deal of time with Tony Ownbey, whose younger brother, Tim, had died in Vietnam from a land mine explosion just a few months earlier. The Ownbey family struggled greatly over Tim's death. His passing touched the hearts of many in the Eugene/Springfield area.

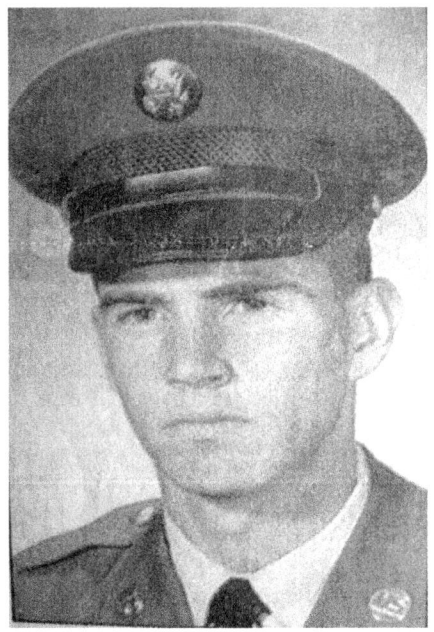

Tim Ownbey (1969 or 1970)

Author and Eugene's *The Register-Guard* columnist Bob Welch, in his book *A Father for all Seasons* (Harvest House, 1998), devoted two chapters describing the unique relationship between Tim, Larry, and their fathers, both named Jay. Welch mentions that the two Jays served in the Navy during World War II. They were the same age. The sons, close friends, also the same age, served in Vietnam. The Brownings and Ownbeys were native North Carolinians who moved to Washington, and then Oregon. And both families suffered tragic loss within two months of each other.

Welch tells of Tim's honorable service in Vietnam. He earned a Bronze Star for an attempted rescue of a downed pilot. A shoulder wound from a Viet Cong bullet sent him to a South China Sea hospital, perhaps the same one where Larry had convalesced. Tim recovered from the gunshot and returned to combat, only to be killed by the land-mine explosion.

1970, possibly the worst year of Larry's life, finally ended. The days of January passed by and Larry prepared for his return to Vietnam.

Then he received some surprising news. The Army "compassionately reassigned" him to Fort Lewis, Washington. Oddly enough, Larry would have preferred returning to Vietnam. The Fort Lewis assignment, though safe, required that he serve an additional four months. "As a pathfinder [in Vietnam], I had a pretty secure job. There wasn't a lot of chance of being attacked or anything."

At Fort Lewis, he began working at the Basic Training Committee Group. The Army promoted him to corporal and he performed odd jobs such as setting up and taking down weapons at the firing range. He also became a chauffeur of sorts, driving the sergeant major and colonel around the post. He drove new officers around in a large bus and dropped them off at the officers club for drinks. Larry spent a lot of time waiting in vehicles and reading newspapers.

One day, the sergeant major approached Larry and said, "Browning, you've been promoted to sergeant." A pay raise and added responsibilities accompanied the promotion. Larry became a "compass and pace" instructor, and put his pathfinder's skills to good use. He taught trainees how to navigate unfamiliar terrain. Larry would send them out on a simulation course for an hour, and review their findings when they returned. Some of his pupils were officers.

One day, a lieutenant performed badly on the pace course and accused Larry of giving him inadequate instructions.

Larry told the officer, "If you would have been paying attention, you would have known what you should have done."

The steamed lieutenant said, "You can't talk to me that way."

"Well, sir," responded Sergeant Browning, "as long as you're on my compass course, I have authority over you. And if I want to, I can kick you off. So if you feel like you need to go talk to my commanding officer, you go right ahead."

"Well," said the lieutenant, "we'll see about that." He promptly presented his grievance to the colonel. The colonel backed Larry and advised the humbled lieutenant to start listening to his instructor.

Larry spent most of his time at Fort Lewis running the compass and pace courses. During that time, a major and a sergeant first class tried to persuade him to reenlist, but he refused, figuring they'd send him back to Vietnam.

"I decided to apply for an early out," says Larry. "And so that came through. I got out September 17th, 1971."

The twenty-one year old received his honorable discharge—but not without a hitch.

The war would haunt him for the rest of his life.

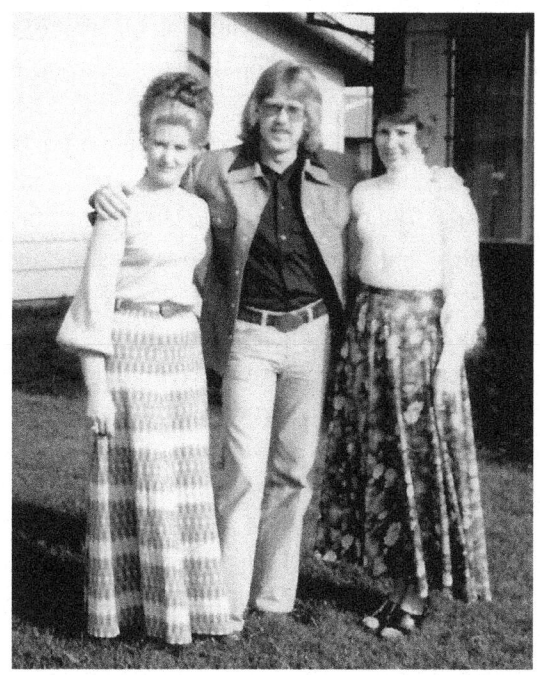

Larry with mother Agatha and sister Brenda. 1970's

ഇൻൽ

7

WANDER YEARS

These days Larry's adventures consist of being rolled from one part of the house to the other. Long naps fill the gaps between rides. This is the routine. Though he's not happy with this existence, Larry has learned to be content.

Attending church on Sunday mornings provides a nice change of pace from the weekday repetition. But it's more than that. Larry experiences significant joy and meaning from church.

He places the utmost value on the gathering together of the body of Christ for worship and fellowship. Relationships mean everything to him.

But it's midweek and another humdrum morning. I roll Larry into the kitchen and park him beside the dining table. Breakfast is his favorite meal of the day. He prefers Total Raisin Bran, but it's fairly high in calories, so today he opts for something low-cal.

"I'll have Special K and a banana."

Larry's caloric intake must be kept to a bare minimum or he gains weight. His metabolism runs incredibly slow because his only exercise comes from jaw movement needed to eat and talk.

He's learned to be content with a small amount of food.

I empty one cup of Special K into a bowl, add sliced bananas, sprinkle some stevia sweetener over it, and pour in one-half cup of watery-looking skim milk. This is his typical breakfast. On rare occasions, he'll splurge and eat something fatty, such as bacon and eggs.

After pouring his coffee, I steal a cup for myself. Then I sit down and spoon bite after bite of cereal into his mouth.

I ask him how he's able to be content when he's physically restricted in nearly every area of his life. Larry explains, "He [God] puts you in circumstances where you can either learn contentment or not. It's kind of like an exercise on building your faith."

He chews a spoonful of cereal and says that a contented attitude is not automatic for Christians. It doesn't just happen, but is learned through hardship. Then he mentions the good news: "I can do all things *through* Christ who strengthens me." He's referring to Philippians 4:12-13 where the Apostle Paul writes, "…I have learned the secret of being content in any and every situation, whether well fed or hungry, whether living in plenty or in want. I can do everything through Him who gives me strength."

"So, what do we do to receive that strength?" I ask, hoping to hear a foolproof formula that guarantees God's power in three easy steps.

Larry sucks in some coffee through the taped-on straw. "We need to yield to the Holy Spirit, recognize our weakness, and as Paul said, we need to die daily, put off our selfish ambitions and trust the Lord."

Whew, not so easy.

"But, don't those things you just mentioned also require God's power to do them?" I ask.

Larry pauses, then quotes Colossians 3:2: "Setting our minds on things above, not on things below." He explains, "We get in trouble when we think fleshly and not spiritually. Isaiah 26:3 says, 'You keep him in perfect peace whose mind is stayed on You, because he trusts in You.' It's not easy. At times you have a pity party."

Larry mentions the early years of his ministry when financial difficulties presented the greatest test to his contentment. During the 1980's, when he attended seminary and began his first pastorate in Dorris, California, he and his late wife Karen faced continual financial challenges. They often wondered how they would pay their next bill. The couple continued to pray, tithe and remain faithful.

"Never once did we miss a payment."

I ask if he was discontented during his rebellious years after the war.

"Very discontented," he says and opens his mouth for another bite of Special K.

છ૭ભ

Escape. Larry had seen the horror of war and received an honorable discharge. The twenty one year-old came home to anything but a hero's welcome. The liberal protestors called Vietnam vets baby killers. Hard-nosed conservatives considered them dopers and losers, unable to finish the job of winning a war.

No ticker tape parades for these guys. So Larry did what many other Vietnam vets did at the time: grew his hair long, smoked lots of pot and tried to blend in with the hippie culture prevalent at the time. Most of all, he tried to forget the war. Escape.

Along with his desire to forget, Larry felt genuine joy and excitement at his discharge. "It was kind of a sense of freedom. For two years you were told when to eat, where to go and what to do. Other than the fact that I didn't have any direction in my life, I was looking forward to being separated from the Army."

Larry returned to Oregon from Fort Lewis in the fall of 1971. He and his friend Craig Matsler rented an apartment in Eugene. Their pal Steve Keller soon moved in. These were the same buddies Larry hung out with prior to the war.

The three made a pact not to cut their hair for two years. Steve, with curly locks, grew a big, floppy afro. Craig, who also had curls, developed cascading waves. Larry's straight hair grew the longest—as in halfway down his back. "It was as long as my girlfriend's," he says.

"We were the Three Stooges," says, uh, Larry. "Craig was more like Larry. I was more like Curly. I think Steve [who had curly hair] was Moe." Nothing is as it seems.

All that hair served as a type of camouflage, hiding their identity as war veterans. "Once our hair got long," says Larry, "they thought we were just hippies. They didn't even know we'd been in the service."

A few things had changed for the trio since that brief time between high school and the war. They'd lost any hint of innocence for one thing. But the greatest loss came from the death of Tim Ownbey, who once completed the close-knit group. Two years earlier, the life insurance salesman told the foursome that one in four Vietnam soldiers died in service. The statistic, though inaccurate overall, bore true in the case of these particular friends.

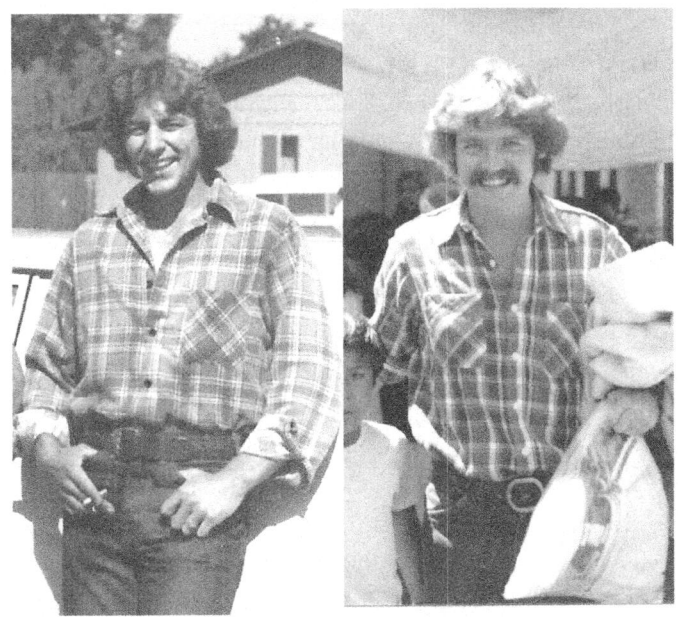

Craig Matsler and Steve Keller, 1970's

Larry's three-month early release from military service came with the stipulation that he enter college immediately. With financial assistance from the G.I. Bill, Larry attended classes at Lane Community College in Eugene. He leaned toward journalism because he liked to write and enjoyed talking to people.

By the end of the school year, his interest waned. "At that time I had started doing drugs, mostly smoking pot. I smoked it every day and had low motivation…and didn't do real well in school."

Larry ditched college in the spring of 1972 and took a job at Weyerhaeuser Lumber Company, where he had worked just before joining the Army. He passed their physical, which in those days didn't include a drug test.

Weyerhaeuser provided a nice benefit for veterans, allowing them to build up seniority while in the service. To the disdain of several employees, Larry, with shoulder length hair (and growing), immediately got one of the good jobs in the planing mill.

"Sometimes at lunchtime we'd go out and smoke a joint. You know, I never could figure out why they didn't smell it on us—maybe it was because we'd smoke a cigarette afterwards. But the job I had didn't take a lot of concentration, so if something happened, the set-up man would go fix it. I'd just kind of stand around."

He was a functional druggie, who could perform job duties well, despite being high morning, noon and night. Marijuana became his bread-and-butter dope. To a lesser degree he used alcohol, speed, mescaline, peyote, cocaine and LSD. Larry hid his substance abuse from those he thought would disapprove. For a few years, his mother was unaware of his lifestyle.

That summer, Larry and some friends attended the Oregon Renaissance Faire, an annual hippie festival later renamed the Oregon Country Fair. It had a reputation as a vortex for pervasive drug use and rampant paganism (though in later years the organizers would discourage the drug use). The iconic psychedelic folk-rock band, the Grateful Dead, played the day Larry visited, and the Free Souls motorcycle gang was hired to keep the crowd under control and off the stage.

The temperature rose to a toasty 103 degrees and water was scarce. Larry nearly suffered from heat exhaustion after taking the hallucinogen mescaline. He found relief when a fire truck arrived and hosed the revelers down. He located a non-alcoholic beverage to quench his thirst, and sat under a shady tree until he recovered enough to resume partying.

Larry quit Weyerhaeuser in the fall of 1972 and reenrolled at Lane Community College. But once again, his studies fizzled from too much pot and lack of ambition. Over the course of three terms, he did manage to earn A's in three writing classes. An interest in poetry stuck and he continued to dabble in verse for several years. At the end of spring term, he returned to Weyerhauser. He worked there a few weeks; then an adventurous job opportunity arose.

In the spring of 1973, Chuck Oliver, the father of Larry's girlfriend, offered Larry an enticing job prospect in Alaska. Oliver, a successful owner of a logging company, decided to move his business to Alaska where he would log and build roads. He needed someone to clean up and renovate an old bunkhouse that would be used to house his employees. He offered the job to Larry, who'd previously earned Oliver's confidence by helping him out on a number of work projects.

"He was just too nice of a guy," says Larry, mentioning that Chuck's kindhearted, trusting spirit resulted in people sometimes taking advantage of him.

Chuck knew Larry had smoked some pot, but the elder didn't realize the extent of it. The entire Oliver family would soon travel north to join Chuck once the business got underway.

Larry, now twenty-three, jumped at the opportunity. "I'd love to go with you," he told Chuck. "When are you leaving?"

"In the morning," said Chuck.

Larry had to give Weyerhaeuser short notice. His crew boss said, "No problem."

Chuck picked Larry up the next morning and they flew from Eugene to Ketchikan. From there they caught a small plane to Wrangell Island in southeastern Alaska. Oliver set up shop in the town of Wrangell, population two thousand.

Larry went to work on the rundown bunkhouse, once used in the 1950's and 60's by Filipinos working at a fish cannery. He replaced 278 wood-framed windows, helped build showers and a laundry room. When he finished cleaning and fixing the place up, Larry made himself a room in the bunkhouse. By then, he and Chuck's daughter were no longer dating.

At the Wrangell Island post office, Larry ran into a fellow Thurston High School graduate named Bud Washerman, a carpenter. The two started hanging out together. Bud approached him one day and proposed they start a remodeling business together. The timing was good, because work had dwindled with Oliver. Bud and Larry became partners and found plenty of jobs.

Larry's daily marijuana habit continued. His connection from Springfield routinely mailed packages of Thai stick, a potent form of pot laced with opium. Larry sold the stuff at twice the cost and became the primary dealer in Wrangell Island.

"I think how stupid I was, because if I'd ever got caught receiving marijuana through the mail, they'd have sent me to federal prison."

Larry needed a new place to stay and rented a bed at a Catholic parish operated by a priest named Father Claude, who performed mass on Sundays and sometimes midweek. Larry noticed effeminate speech patterns and mannerisms in the priest.

One night, as Larry jawed with some of the other lodgers, a renter named Scott walked in with a smirk on his face. He said that Father Claude had just hit on him. Scott told the priest not to try it again or he'd kill him. The renters had a good laugh.

An Elks club member, Father Claude attended monthly meetings where he gorged on steak, played cards all night and drank plenty of booze.

One morning, Larry chatted with the priest while they ate breakfast. The conversation turned to religion. The young renter couldn't resist provoking his landlord.

"Claude," said Larry, "do you actually think you're going to heaven?"

"What do you mean, Larry?"

"Well, you play cards and drink. And you don't just drink a little—you get drunk. Then you come home, get up on Sunday and do mass. You drink *here* all the time too. You don't actually believe you're going to heaven, do ya?"

"Well," answered the cleric, "of course I do."

"Claude," said Larry, "you're going to hell just like the rest of us."

The priest rose from the table and left the room. That evening, when Larry returned home from work, he found a dirty frying pan on his pillow with a note inside that said, *Wash me and be out by morning.* Larry had forgotten to clean his dishes after breakfast.

The next day, Larry packed up his belongings and visited a friend, Greg McCormick, who owned a big three-bedroom trailer. Larry moved in. Greg would become a good, lifelong friend. Years later he became a Christian.

Larry completed his remodeling work with Bud Washerman, and in the fall of 1973 returned to Oregon for a few months to give Lane Community College one more try. He lasted one term and moved back to Wrangell Island that winter. He took a job driving a delivery truck for Greg McCormick, who owned a transfer and storage business.

Larry's time in Alaska lasted about a year and a half. In the fall of 1974 he moved back to Springfield with $2000 in savings. He moved in with his mom and took a lengthy break from work.

At this time, Agatha suspected her son of drug use. She mentioned to him that it seemed odd that he had so many friends going in and out of his bedroom. Though he told her otherwise, Larry was inside selling pot. She never caught him with drugs or found any in his room, but promised him she'd call the police if she ever did.

In February, 1975, Larry and a friend named Hal decided to travel through Mexico for a month. Prior to leaving, they cut their hair, thinking the hippie look would draw unwanted attention from the Mexican police. Carrying backpacks, sleeping bags and plenty of traveler's checks, the gringos took a train across the border. They decided not to bring any pot with them, hoping to score local stuff in Mexico.

The rough, twenty-two hour train ride took them to Mazatlan. They stayed there a week, hung out at the beach, and drank extra booze to compensate for the lack of pot.

A migrant worker, Luis, invited them to travel with him to a carnival near Takolotlan, Jalisco. Like eager pups they said yes, and the next morning hopped into Luis's babied '68 Plymouth Roadrunner.

On the way to the carnival, Luis asked his passengers if they wanted to smoke some pot. The two had endured nearly two weeks without any dope, so they jumped at the opportunity. Luis took a detour into a rocky desert. He stopped the car, walked toward a rock, turned it over and pulled out a bag of marijuana.

Larry and Hal assumed the Mexican weed would be more potent than in the states. Luis rolled a few joints and put the bag back under the rock.

Says Larry, "My thought was, 'How does he know where the rock's at?' There were lots of rocks out there and we were in the middle of nowhere."

The three toked up with less than satisfying results. "Well," says Larry, "it wasn't very good pot. But we didn't say anything."

They arrived for the last day of the weeklong carnival. A bullfight highlighted the afternoon's festivities. A fenced area substituted for an arena and the bulls lacked spirit. The local men tried to persuade the two Americans to get into the ring, but they declined. Instead, Larry took photos.

The festival climaxed that evening with a big dance. A four-piece band, with fur-covered guitars, played a mix of American and Latino music. Larry and Hal wanted to dance, but the language barrier made them timid. Hal knew a few words of Spanish, but not enough for a conversation. So they kept on the sidelines despite encouraging glances from pretty Mexican women.

The Oregon boys continued on through Guadalajara and Mexico City. Their pot habit remained unsated, so they caught a night train to Oaxaca, rumored to be a major hub for potent marijuana.

They arrived in Oaxaca the next day and checked in at a motel. They walked to the town square and scoped out the marketplace. Street musicians played. A restaurant with outdoor seating caught their eyes. They ordered beers and sat down. Beggar children approached and tried to sell them Chiclets. Larry's heart went out to a little boy with a cleft palate and not much nose. He gave the boy some change and more beggars followed. It proved impossible to relax, so they finished their beers and escaped the beggars.

Still longing for a decent high, the pothead duo scoured the city for a bag of weed. "We were in the courtyard," says Larry, "and these two Mexican guys came up to us and we asked them if they had any pot. They said, 'Yeah,' and told us to meet them back there later that evening."

Late that night, Larry and Hal showed up at the designated spot. The two Mexicans arrived and told the Americans to follow them. They walked along dimly lit streets. Larry didn't see any other white people around. He felt uneasy.

The Mexicans entered a motel and beckoned the wary gringos to follow. The four passed by a bored attendant and continued along an empty hallway. They climbed some stairs and passed through another hallway. The Mexicans stopped at a room and opened the door. They motioned the Americans to follow them inside.

"We went into the room where they were staying and we kind of haggled with them and decided how much we wanted. Then they left the room. I'm thinking: *these guys could rob us or kill us*. I told Hal, 'If something happens, don't worry about me. It's every man for himself.'"

The two Mexicans returned to the room and pulled out a quarter pound bag of marijuana. The Americans paid five dollars for it, an incredibly cheap price. With the deal secured, Larry and Hal hit the street and hustled away, making sure the dealers were out of sight. When they returned to their motel room, they cleaned the pot, picking out the undesirable stems and seeds.

Their stress level increased because of the constant effort required to keep the stuff concealed. They knew full well, if caught, a rough Mexican jail awaited them. Each day, the two alternated who held the pot. This way, only the carrier would be arrested and jailed. The other could then try to pay off the police for his friend's freedom. "When I carried it," says Larry, "I stuck it in my boot and pulled my pants down over it. I don't know what Hal did with it."

The high-quality grass enabled them to stay stoned for the rest of the trip. The Mexican adventure, which also included some legitimate sightseeing, lasted a month and only cost them about six hundred dollars each.

Back home and unemployed, Larry scoured the newspaper for jobs and started selling life insurance in the summer of 1975. A bout with pneumonia kept him in bed for a month. He recovered and resumed door-to-door sales, but felt guilty pushing policies on low-income elderly folks. He quit after a few months.

Larry worked for a short time building home foundations, then took a truck-driving job hauling bark mulch and other forest byproducts. He continued to party, hang out at bars and smoke marijuana daily through most of 1976. Several out-of-state road trips kept his wanderlust in check.

1976 marked a turning point for Larry. Near the end of the year, he started to evaluate his life for the first time since high school. "Here I was at age twenty-six and I realized I didn't have any sense of purpose in my life. I began to think of the calling I had when I was eighteen."

Having lived with roommates for the last eight years, Larry decided to find a place by himself. He rented a duplex in Springfield and began to distance himself from his druggie friends. He stopped drinking and hanging out at bars, but continued to smoke pot daily.

In March of 1977 he took a mill job at Rosboro Lumber Company and settled into a daily grind of work, eat, sleep and marijuana use. To break the monotony he bought a sweet '64

Corvette Roadster. On the Fourth of July weekend, he and Craig Matsler cruised north on I-5 toward Seattle. They took a detour in Vancouver and visited a friend named Dennis, whose girlfriend had a friend named Karen Adams. Dennis insisted that Larry meet Karen. Larry obliged, always happy to meet a new babe. She dropped by later that day.

"I thought she was kind of attractive," says Larry.

Romantic fireworks were apparently limited to sparklers that day. After all, it was just the third of July.

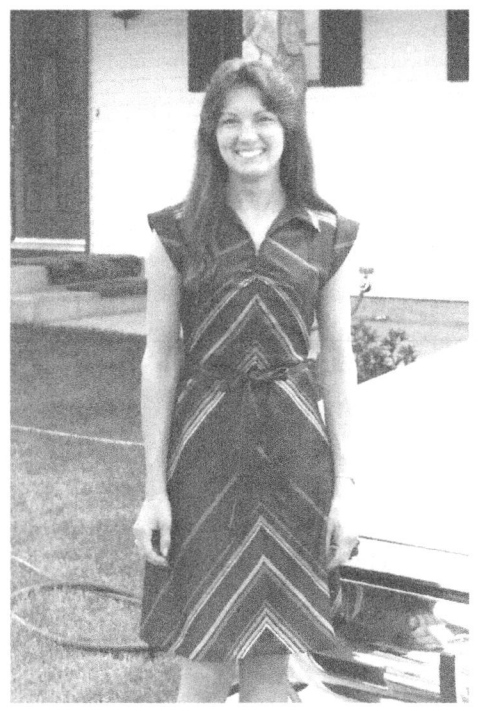

Karen (1978 or 79)

৪০৫৩

8

THE PRODIGAL SON RETURNS

Larry's hospice nurse, Margie, arrives at the house. She visits every other week. I'm off the clock, waiting at the dining room table until Larry's freed up to do another interview. He and Margie chat in the living room about meds, blood pressure, shoulder pain and, yes, boogers. Lately, there's been extra buildup in his nostrils. Larry can't simply grab a tissue and blow his nose. And even when someone else holds the tissue against his nostrils, his breath is so weak that he can't adequately blow out mucous. One must twist tissues into reamers and clean out each nostril. It's one more discomfort to add to his list.

The Christmas tree is up and boxes of ornaments sit on the floor. Ann enters the living room and apologizes for the holiday clutter. She joins the conversation with Larry and Margie.

It's December 18, 2010 and Larry has been on hospice since September. At that time the neurologist said he'd probably live up to a year. His ability to swallow will likely be the next thing to go. Larry has it in writing that he does not want to have a feeding tube. If he doesn't contract a respiratory illness that stops his already weak breathing, it's likely he will die from starvation.

He's not worried though, having endured worse pain already. When God chooses to take him home, he knows the release will be good.

But I will miss him very much.

The session ends. Margie gathers her things and says goodbye. I enter the living room and ask Larry if he's ready for the interview.

"You bet," he says.

Ann resumes decorating. Larry and I get out of her way, moving to the dining table next to the kitchen. She's within earshot of us. Most of the questions will focus on Larry's late wife Karen.

Ann and Larry's daughter, Paige, just arrived home from fall classes at California Baptist University in Riverside. She's off getting a haircut. Paige is Karen and Larry's daughter by birth.

I turn on the recorder and ask Larry a few mundane questions about names, places and dates. Then I clear my throat. "I'd like to switch to some questions about Karen."

"Yeah," says Larry.

I turn and face the living room, "Is that okay with you, Ann?"

"Yeah." Ann is generally straightforward and speaks her mind honestly—so I take her at her word. She's fine with the subject of Larry's previous wife.

Larry is a guy's guy who lavishes more details about his '64 Corvette Roadster than the emotions he felt during his courtship with and marriage to Karen. My questions are decidedly touchy-feely, often beginning with the four words, "How did you feel…?" Larry endures the grilling, but sometimes I feel like I'm pulling teeth.

We move through the early romance to the darker time when they separated. The critical issue concerned Larry's marijuana habit. Karen refused to put up with it and verbally harangued him whenever she found him stoned, which was almost daily.

As Larry tells me this, I'm thinking, *You go girl! Hit him hard and don't let up until he quits.* I figure intervention is essential in these situations.

But Larry sees it differently. "The thing I kept telling Karen was, 'Quit playing the role of the Holy Spirit.' I was [already] being convicted [by God] and her getting upset with me didn't help at all because it made me want to just resist more and more."

I try to see his side. "Well, that's sort of biblical, about the unbelieving husband and the believing wife. She's to be silent and win him with her goodness." I'm thinking along the lines of 1 Peter 3:1-2.

Ann walks into the kitchen. "You know, Larry, you've never been in the reverse situation."

"No, I haven't," he grants.

I perk up, hoping Ann elaborates. But she humbly opts

out and returns to the living room. She need not say more, because Larry and I are quite aware that in her previous marriage Ann suffered a "reverse situation" and worse. At that time, escape was her best option, not silence.

The Q&A continues, covering humdrum stuff such as mortgages and 7% GI loans. Then I ask if Karen ever admitted being too hard on him about his pot habit.

"No," he answers, "not that I can remember."

As we progress through the interview, it becomes clear that Karen was an attractive, strong-willed and stubborn woman. These traits caused Larry some frustration, but it should be mentioned that, ultimately, her stubborn perseverance saved their marriage.

The questions cease and I'm dissatisfied. Larry didn't say what I wanted him to say. It seems disrespectful to the memory of Karen for him to insist that her heated exhortations for him to quit using pot were in vain. But Larry speaks it the way he sees it, not the way I think it should be. Life is unpredictable—and messy.

So, how did he find the mettle to quit smoking dope? Larry claims that one day, out of the blue, the sovereign God of the universe intervened and instantly took away his desire for marijuana and tobacco. He says it was a miracle from heaven.

God did it, not Karen.

I think of Larry's current sufferings and I want them to somehow impact me, move me to great change. But after a year and a half as his caregiver, I'm still the same person with the same struggles. Sure, I've gained wisdom from Larry's life and words—and wisdom reflects maturity. But has real change occurred in my heart and actions? I'm not sure.

Then it hits me. Larry is not the Holy Spirit. There's nothing he can say, there's no amount of suffering he can endure that will result in one ounce of change in my heart.

Only God can do that.

৳০৩

Larry's walk with God followed a path similar to his courtship and marriage to Karen Adams. Both relationships progressed through love, separation, reconciliation and healing.

When Larry and Karen met on July 3, 1977, it wasn't love at first sight. Sure, he found her attractive—a brunette with long, flowing hair and deeply tanned skin. But the initial encounter was brief.

A day later, Larry joined Karen and four others for the Fourth of July drag races at Portland International Raceway. The group consisted of three men and three women. They'd barely found seats in the stands when the three guys took off to a nearby hillside to smoke pot. When they returned to their seats, Karen appeared embarrassed and a bit shocked by their brazen marijuana use. Not much conversation happened during the races.

Afterwards, Larry, 27, drove Karen, 21, back to Vancouver in his Corvette. The four others rode in another vehicle. A traffic jam made it a long drive and Larry tried to use the numerous stops to his advantage. With one goal on his mind, he sweet-talked Karen as best he could. She stayed fairly quiet as he blathered on. At one point, he leaned over and kissed her. She allowed it, but only one.

"Later on," says Larry, "she told me that she thought I was too forward and she kind of said to herself, *What does he think he's doing?"*

He dropped her off at her apartment. They said goodnight, and their first date ended. In essence, Larry made a bad first impression, thanks to his pot smoking and dishonorable intentions.

Why Karen continued to see him mystifies Larry. "The only thing I know is I had a Corvette and I wasn't bad looking."

The day after that first date, Larry and Craig Matsler headed south on I-5 back to Springfield. During the drive, the Corvette began vibrating, and they pulled off the freeway. The lug nuts had loosened on a wheel, reaming out the rim. They hitchhiked to the nearest rest area, called several friends and asked if they'd pick them up. No one said yes. Larry resorted to calling his mom. Agatha came through and rescued her boy. The next day, Larry and Craig returned with a trailer and hauled the car back to Springfield.

"I had to buy all new rims for my Corvette," says Larry, "which turned out to be a good thing. It really looked nice."

Over the next few months, Karen and Larry visited each other most weekends. This required that one or the other endure the two-and-a-half hour drive between Springfield and Vancouver—a five-hour round trip. Karen visited Larry more than he visited her.

During this time, Larry made no effort to hide his marijuana habit. He didn't perceive any disapproval from Karen, who didn't smoke pot.

Both were romantically attracted to each other, but Larry had previously been attracted to other women as well. Romance may have been Karen's motivation to pursue the relationship, but something else drove Larry.

They'd discovered at the outset a mutual faith in Christ, though both were immature believers. Despite his compromised lifestyle, Larry knew he wanted to marry a Christian. Karen's faith was genuine. She came to know the Lord despite her unbelieving parents' negative influence.

"You know," says Larry, "I believe the bottom line is that God was in the mix, and in a sense God ordained that relationship because if it had been fleshly, I don't think I'd ever have married her."

The couple never sought premarital counseling, and if they had, Larry wouldn't have admitted his vices to the counselor. He acknowledges that "any kind of a good pastor" would have advised Karen against marrying him.

Four months after they met, Larry proposed to her in Vancouver on Thanksgiving Day, 1977. They'd gone for a leisurely drive after eating a turkey dinner with her family. He parked the Corvette and popped the big question. She said yes.

They exchanged vows at Karen's church in Vancouver on March 3, 1978. She wore her older sister Patti's wedding dress, white with a short train. Her best friend, Diane Wilson, was maid of honor. Her sisters, Patti, Sharon, Diane and Michelle, were bridesmaids. Larry, hair now at shoulder length, wore a white tux. Craig Matsler served as best man. The groomsmen were Steve Keller and Dennis Lynch.

The newlyweds enjoyed a three-day honeymoon at the central Oregon resort, Sunriver. Larry couldn't squeeze any more time than that off work.

They moved into Larry's duplex in Springfield. Karen found a job as a secretary and he continued at Rosboro Lumber. They purchased a home. Larry had enough saved for the down payment.

As weeks turned to months, each person's true colors emerged. Larry continued to smoke pot daily. He had entered the marriage assuming Karen didn't mind, but her annoyance soon surfaced. She began to confront him about his habit. He resisted. Tensions increased. They argued as often as she found him stoned.

Ironically, as their marriage worsened, Larry's thoughts focused more and more on God. This slow move back to Christ had begun about a year before meeting Karen. In 1976 he had stopped hanging out at bars and began to reflect on the calling he'd felt at age eighteen. Heart changes were now happening, but without much visible evidence.

Karen saw a man with a daily marijuana habit, who defiantly resisted change.

But in his heart and mind, Larry felt something else. "The Holy Spirit was convicting me that I needed to quit [smoking pot], but Karen just ragged on me all the time."

The verbal brawls worsened. After a year and a half of marriage, they'd had enough.

"We decided to go our separate ways," says Larry.

In September of 1979, Karen packed up most of her possessions and moved back to Vancouver. Larry remained in the Springfield home.

A friend named Ray Lodeen moved in. This helped lighten the mortgage payments. Ray had recently recommitted his life to the Lord.

Despite the setback of a failed marriage, Larry continued taking steps toward God. He now prayed regularly for the Lord to deliver him from his marijuana habit. He and Ray started going to church, trying out a new one each week. They attended four different churches in four weeks. "Every time I walked into a church, the pastor was preaching on divorce. So I really felt some deep conviction. But at the same time, I was still very stubborn and rebellious."

He called Karen a few times during the first and second months of separation to attempt reconciliation. Each time, she responded by asking if he had quit smoking pot. He said no—so she said no. By the third month, he lost all desire to reunite with her.

At four months Larry filed for divorce. He mailed the

papers to Karen, requesting her signature. The deal stated she could have everything but the house.

A few days later Karen called and said she didn't want to divorce. She felt they hadn't given their marriage a chance. She wanted to come down that weekend and discuss getting back together.

"I told her that I didn't want to continue the relationship and didn't love her anymore, that...all she had to do was sign them [the papers] and we'd be divorced. Karen, being more stubborn than I am, said that she was coming down to visit me. I told her I didn't want her to come down."

He also told her he had a date set up with another woman and didn't want to break it. She said, "Well, I'm coming anyway."

Larry canceled his date and Karen arrived at the door as promised. He let her inside and they talked. She made clear her desire to give their marriage another try.

"I was very honest with her and said that I'd really lost all feelings of love toward her."

Though he felt no love, he did feel intense conviction from the Holy Spirit. The recent sermons against divorce still lingered fresh in his mind. God's will became clear. At some point during the conversation, Larry relented and agreed to reunite. He made no promises to quit his pot habit and she backed off on that point. Mission accomplished, Karen drove back to Vancouver and gathered her belongings. She quickly returned and moved back in.

"I committed to get back together, not because I had any feelings of love toward her, but because I had made a commitment to God," says Larry. "So many people today want to divorce because they say they have irreconcilable differences, but when you take your marriage vows, you say for better or worse, in sickness and in health, for richer or poorer, till death do we part."

His reconciliation with Karen was actually a step of obedience to God and a significant step toward his rededication to the Lord. In 1980, the couple began attending Trinity Baptist Church in Springfield, where Larry went as a boy with his family. His mother, Agatha, and her second husband, Lynn Morse, were currently members there.

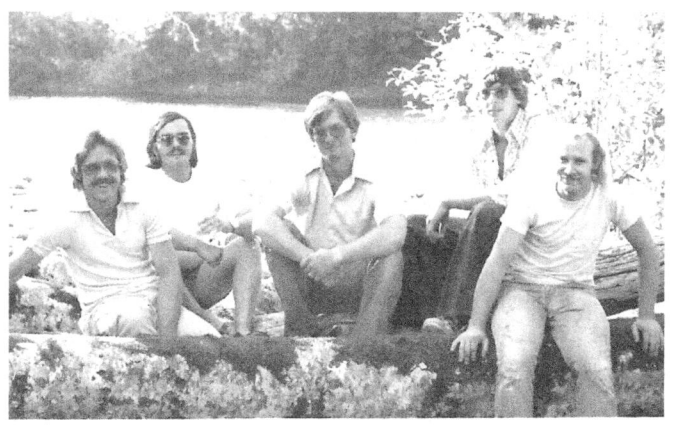

Larry and fellow members of the band *Destiny.* 1980

Larry and some other guys from Trinity formed a Christian rock band called Destiny. Larry played rhythm electric guitar and sang lead vocals. He'd been playing guitar for eight years. Two other guitarists, a bass player and drummer rounded out the band. They performed at the University of Oregon's student union and a few local churches. The band stayed together a little over two years.

The group had good intentions, but a certain glitch held them back. All of them smoked pot. They rationalized that since marijuana was "natural," it wasn't a sin to use it. Larry halfheartedly went along with that argument. Though he reflects fondly about his time with the band, he acknowledges they probably failed to do much good for the kingdom of God. "I think if we hadn't been smoking pot, we might have actually become more influential."

Larry no longer used marijuana on a daily basis. This resulted in fewer clashes with Karen. She had returned to the marriage knowing full well his hesitancy to recommit. So, pressuring him to quit pot would only push him away. In essence, Larry held the cards. She could make few demands. Of course, the marital strain continued.

As 1980 came to an end, an old stirring resurfaced in Larry's heart. "I really felt God had not taken His call off my life for full-time ministry." He saw the need for Bible training and wanted to pursue an Associate of Divinity Degree at Golden Gate Baptist Theological Seminary. Karen opposed the idea, largely because he still smoked pot. She also felt uneasy about becoming a pastor's wife.

Larry charged ahead with his dream and put their house on the market, even though he hadn't yet applied for admission at Golden Gate. The recession hit at that time and the house didn't sell. It seemed God used the recession to shut the door on Larry's plans for ministry.

"I think until I gave up smoking pot, God wasn't going to allow me to go anywhere."

Larry made several efforts to quit at this time. A cycle occurred where he would buy a bag of weed, smoke a joint, feel convicted and flush the rest down the toilet. The expensive cycle repeated several times. He continued to pray for deliverance.

During 1981, Larry took another step toward God by severing his relationship with his pot-smoking friends. "I told my friends that I couldn't be around them anymore because I wasn't a strong enough Christian not to be tempted by what they were doing."

Then, on January 16, 1982, God instantly took away Larry's desire for both marijuana and tobacco. It was not a disciplined act of willpower. He hadn't planned to quit on that particular day. God simply delivered him.

According to a Psychology Today article by Jann Gumbiner, Ph.D. (December, 2010), about nine percent of regular marijuana users become seriously addicted to the drug, and "…withdrawal symptoms might include: anxiety, depression, nausea, sleep disturbances and gastrointestinal problems." The article states that "…nicotine is much more addictive. It is much harder to quit smoking cigarettes than it is to quit smoking pot."

So it could be argued that the greater miracle was how Larry no longer craved tobacco. He ceased both habits cold turkey, with no withdrawal symptoms. Larry had smoked a pack daily right up until the day he stopped. In thirteen years of smoking tobacco, he'd never tried to quit and had no desire to.

"I liked to smoke," he says.

Oddly enough, a day or two passed before he recognized the miracle. God had performed the healing without fireworks or high drama. Larry simply awoke that morning without a desire to light up.

"I think His timing was good," says Larry, "because He gave me a full eight months that I didn't smoke anything before I went to seminary."

The nasty pot habit had been a ball and chain preventing him from pursuing effective ministry. With the besetting sin gone, doors of God's favor began to open for the first time.

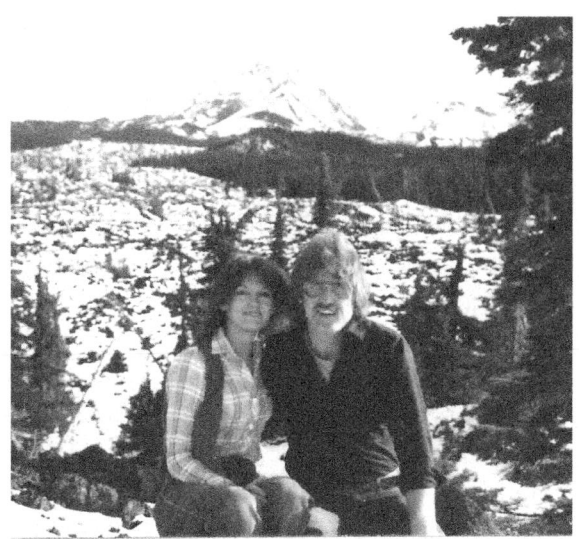

Karen and Larry near the Three Sisters, 1981

☙❧

9

IT IS WELL WITH MY SOUL

Larry's diaphragm is out of shape because he sits motionless day after day. Therefore his breathing is weak and his voice lacks volume. He can only speak a few words with each small breath, often pausing mid-sentence to inhale. Then he finishes the sentence. If some breath remains, he'll start the next sentence without a pause. For the listener, this may create a sense of discontinuity.

At first I mistook the pauses for mental lapses where he tries to gather thoughts before continuing. In the written transcripts of his taped interviews, the pauses between sentences are not visible. When read, Larry's words are clear, fluid, highly detailed and organized. True, the pile of daily meds can make him groggy, and he often naps during the day. But in his mind are a lifetime of vivid memories. And in his heart, a passion burns.

Breakfast is over and I wheel Larry back to his bedroom for a half-hour session on the standing frame, a therapeutic apparatus that enables him to "stand" upright. Using a built-in jack, I crank him up and out of the wheelchair until he's vertical. Two straps, wrapped around his body, secure him to the frame. The standing frame may help improve circulation, maintain bone density, prevent constipation, help the lungs expand, and prevent bed sores. If nothing else, it gives Larry a break from sitting.

"Can you get out the *Amazing Grace* CD?" he asks.

"You bet," I say and flip through the music until I find the requested CD, which contains several old hymns. After placing the disc in the small portable player, I press the start button.

"Put on my headphones, if you will."

"Oh yeah, sorry." I'm supposed to put on Larry's headphones first, before pressing start.

"More volume."

"Okay." I turn it up. "Is that enough?"

"A little more."

I up it more.

"More," he says and shuts his eyes. "There, that's good."

"Good?"

"Yeah."

"I'll go do chores."

He nods. I inspect his posture. His torso wants to tilt a little to one side. I adjust a strap so his upper body is centered.

While Larry's in the standing frame, I make the bed, wipe down the shower and start to clean the kitchen. As I load the dishwasher, I hear his weak, intermittent voice from the bedroom.

He's singing along to a song from the CD, but it's not the hymn *Amazing Grace*. It's the first time I've heard him sing.

"When peace like a river… [breath] …sorrows like sea billows… [breath]…"

His short breaths prevent him from keeping pace with the CD.

"Whatever my lot…it is well…with my soul."

I wonder if Larry's making a declaration of dogged faith in the face of tribulation. Or is he experiencing God's assurance that his soul is well? Maybe it's both. Either way, his efforts at worship touch my heart. My eyes water.

Though Larry is sick in body, his soul thrives in the pinnacle of health.

৪১৩

Larry experienced a personal revival after God healed him of his pot and tobacco addictions. He hungered for God's Word and read the Bible for two to three hours every morning. Significant spiritual growth occurred and his desire to enter full-time ministry intensified.

Not surprisingly, his relationship with Karen improved markedly. They argued less often and their love for each other grew. They disagreed, though, when Larry mentioned his intent to apply for admission at Golden Gate Baptist Theological Seminary in Mill Valley, California. Karen made clear her desire not to be a pastor's wife. But Larry felt certain of his calling and applied for admission. She eventually resigned herself to the idea.

Golden Gate accepted Larry's application. This boosted his spirits and helped confirm his calling. He and Karen decided to keep their Springfield house as a rental while they lived in California. Unfortunately this would add extra stress to their lives due to a series of bad renters. Despite the hassle, they managed to make every mortgage payment until the house sold nine years later.

In August of 1982, eight months after God delivered him from chemical addiction, Larry, thirty-two, moved with Karen to Mill Valley. The seminary overlooked its namesake, the Golden Gate Bridge, about seven miles away.

"We lived in an apartment complex with other couples who had no children."

Karen quickly landed a secretarial job and Larry cleaned offices for a while. He then found work as an all-purpose maintenance man on a large property owned by a wealthy retired couple. Word got around and other offers came in for his quality handyman services. It got to be too much. Eventually, Larry found a good job with regular hours at a moving and storage company based in San Francisco. He worked there throughout his stay at seminary.

Classes began in the fall and Larry faced a full load of coursework. His previous attempts at higher education had flopped, despite the undemanding requirements of a community college. He soon discovered that the academic standards at Golden Gate were much loftier than those of a public junior college.

"In one class alone I had three forty-page papers to do in one semester."

Larry met the challenge, studied hard and earned decent grades. His sharp memory helped, as did the biblical knowledge gained from countless childhood Sunday school classes. Bottom line: he did well on tests without the luxury of adequate study time. He would eventually graduate with an Associate of Divinity degree, earning a 3.25 GPA. Not bad, considering the abuse he had inflicted on his brain from twelve years of dope-smoking.

The intense workload resulted in some mental fatigue, but his life now reflected maturity and purpose. Larry's favorite class was taught by Baker James Cauthen, retired missionary to China and former executive director of the Southern Baptist Convention's Foreign Mission Board. The course covered the Biblical basis for missions, from Genesis to Revelation.

Larry and Karen attended Ygnacio Valley Baptist Church in Walnut Creek. He also found time to attend a discipleship group at the home of Professor Cauthen.

At the end of Larry's first semester, Harry Howard, the chaplain at San Quentin Penitentiary visited the seminary and presented a ministry opportunity to the students. Every Tuesday night, a team of volunteers split into pairs and visited inmates in the lockdown units, known as North Seg. Prisoners in these units did time for serious crimes such as murder and rape.

"They were the worst of the worst," says Larry. These inmates lived under the highest security, spending twenty-three hours of each day in their cells, with only one hour to stretch outside in the yard.

Larry eagerly volunteered. The prison was only a ten minute drive from the seminary. "The first night I went out, I wasn't scared, but a little bit unsure what it would be like. I learned right off the bat that these guys were eager to talk to you because they always wanted to talk to somebody on the outside."

After a few months visiting inmates in North Seg, Larry befriended the chaplain who oversaw San Quentin's east block— death row. Larry switched to death row and began visiting prisoners there once a week. He paired up with another volunteer and the two ministered all day at the prison.

"I was able to lead one gentleman to Christ while I was there," says Larry. "I baptized him in a big tank outside the chapel. It wasn't heated. They brought him out and unshackled him. He got into the tank with me and I baptized him. His name was Keith. After his conversion, he said, 'Larry, if this [death penalty] is what it took to bring me to the Lord, I'm glad that it happened.'"

Later, the courts overturned Keith's conviction and released him from prison. Larry had believed in his innocence all along.

Others were far from innocent. The notorious mass murderer and cult leader, Charles Manson, occupied a cell that Larry walked past before entering death row. Manson, a lifer, had recently been transferred there. "He wouldn't turn his lights on," says Larry. "Occasionally you'd catch a glimpse of him, but he didn't really want to talk to anybody."

During his ministry to death-row inmates, Larry changed his position on capital punishment. His compassion for the prisoners moved him to oppose the death penalty. Later, he would revert to his original stance, favoring the death penalty in some circumstances.

In addition to visiting prison inmates, Larry pursued other ministries as well. Toward the end of his second year at Golden Gate, he volunteered as a youth pastor at Ygnacio Valley Baptist Church where he and Karen attended.

After graduating from Golden Gate in December of 1984, he and Karen moved to Concord, California in the east Bay Area. Larry received an offer for a paid youth pastorate at a young startup church located in Benicia, California. He liked the pastor—a gifted preacher with charisma. Larry accepted the position, which paid $600 per month. He continued working full-time for a moving and storage company where he'd been employed since graduation.

At the Benicia church, Larry worked with a Sunday evening youth group of about ten kids. After a few weeks, the pastor criticized Larry for low numbers, claiming he could have recruited over a hundred kids if he were youth pastor. Larry responded by saying, "Yeah, if all you want to do is entertain them, I could probably have a hundred kids too, but I'm trying to teach them something to help them grow in their relationship with Christ."

When Larry had been at Benicia about six months, the pastor partnered with a realtor and decided to buy a nice old mansion. They hoped to convert it into a church. Somebody from the congregation suggested it would be great for weddings. They agreed and a debate began over whether alcohol should be allowed during receptions. Larry and a friend spoke up against the idea, saying it would be a stumbling block for weak Christians and a bad witness to unbelievers. The members voted. Larry and his friend were the only ones opposed. The two decided to quit the church that night.

He and Karen decided to return to Ygnacio Valley Baptist, where they'd developed a good relationship with the pastor and congregation. Larry was ordained at Ygnacio just after graduation.

Meanwhile, Larry continued once a week with the death-row ministry at San Quentin. Prison ministry inspired him and he felt it could easily become his primary calling. He applied for an area director's position with Prison Fellowship, the ministry founded by Chuck Colson. Larry received a call for an extensive interview in San Francisco. Several other interviewees were present. Larry didn't get the job because he lacked management experience.

He sent out resumes for pastorate positions and remained faithful to his weekly visits to San Quentin. Volunteerism didn't pay the bills, so Larry worked various jobs while seeking career ministry opportunities. Since graduation he had worked full-time for Allied Van Lines, a job that lasted a year and a half. In 1986 he worked briefly for another moving company, then found a job driving an eighteen-wheeler that hauled steel to military installations in Sacramento.

In August of 1986, Larry received a response to one of his resumes. First Baptist Church in Dorris, California needed a new pastor. They asked him to visit and preach a sample sermon to the tiny congregation of seventeen.

He, Karen and two friends drove there on a Saturday. "It was high desert, beautiful country," says Larry. "Mount Shasta kind of shadowed over it." They attended a church potluck that evening and spent the night at a member's house. The next morning, Larry preached. He felt a little nervous, having only preached a few times to adults as a youth pastor.

"It went pretty well," he recalls.

After the service, Larry, Karen and the two friends took a long route home, visiting Reno and Carson City along the way. When they arrived back at the Bay Area, a message awaited them on their answering machine. The voice of a Dorris member, Lee Harrington, said the congregation had decided by a vote of fifteen to two, to call Larry as their pastor.

He'd find out later that the two dissenters had voted against him as an act of mercy. They felt if the young pastor were hired, he'd be entering a lion's den. The tiny congregation suffered from petty divisions.

Unaware of these problems, Larry returned Lee's call and said he needed a week to pray about it before deciding. Part of him wanted to say yes immediately, but he felt reservations due to the town's location. "Dorris, California was kind of on the backside of nowhere," says Larry.

He and Karen prayed about it for a week and felt the Lord directing them there. Larry called Lee and asked about salary. The news hurt. The tiny church could only pay four hundred dollars a month and cover rent. Larry and Karen would need to find other jobs for their primary income.

"But we really felt it was God's will for us," says Larry, "so we accepted."

On September 1, 1986, the Brownings moved to Dorris, California, population one-thousand. So began a new phase of Larry's life—pastor of First Baptist Church in Smalltown, USA.

His congregation at Dorris consisted mostly of folks over sixty. He and Karen moved into a "cute…little doll house," as he describes it. Inefficient wall heaters resulted in unexpectedly high electric bills. Karen found a job at a doctor's office and Larry worked various odd jobs.

His first pastorate lacked a honeymoon period. The congregation had been feuding over a frivolous issue weeks before Larry arrived. No one gave him a heads-up. The problem began when the church treasurer decided to set up a fund for a new piano. The church's sole deacon and self-proclaimed manager, opposed the fund because the treasurer hadn't sought approval from the church members. The congregation had divided over the issue and they decided to put it to a vote at the upcoming monthly business meeting. Larry, only a few weeks into his job, would preside.

Official members of First Baptist could vote—including those who rarely attended church. So the lone deacon got on the phone and convinced several AWOL members to attend the meeting and vote against the fund. His opposition did likewise—in favor of the fund. Thirty-two members showed up to vote, despite the fact that only seventeen of them regularly attended church.

After a heated discussion, Larry called for a vote. "When the ballots were counted," says Larry, "it was sixteen for, and sixteen against—which meant, as moderator, I had to make the final decision."

Larry told them he needed a week to think and pray about it. Around midweek, the treasurer approached him and said, "Pastor Larry, I'm really sorry that you got caught in between this. I'll just withdraw my motion to buy a piano [from a church fund]."

In the end, the treasurer simply donated a piano privately to the church. The deacon wasn't thrilled at the outcome, but no rule existed that prohibited private donations. So he conceded, albeit with clenched teeth.

Larry visited members of First Baptist who had stopped attending and asked them why. One fellow said, "Yeah, I'm a member down there, but I'm not ever coming back."

Larry asked, "Well, why not?"

The man answered, "Because all those people do down there is argue and fight."

He never did return to church, but as the months passed by, other past members began attending again.

Divisiveness diminished. In fact, the members unified around one cause—the need to attract young people to the church. Larry naturally embraced the task.

"The only strategy was to love people," he says, "and I really became a part of the local community." He volunteered at Dorris's Butte Valley High School, where he coached JV basketball, JV football, and varsity baseball.

Larry found steady work as an all-purpose man at a large ranch. He and Karen moved into a nice doublewide trailer located on the ranch. The rent was low and it had a wood stove, which reduced their heating bill.

First Baptist began to grow. A youth group formed and grew to about eighteen or twenty kids. They met in the

Brownings' trailer. Troubled kids with neglectful, drug-abusing parents, spent lots of time with Larry and Karen. "There were a couple of the girls that even considered Karen their mom because their [real] moms were off into drugs."

In addition to her ministry to troubled children, Karen taught Sunday school for kids aged six through twelve. Larry taught the teenagers. Vacation Bible School drew nearly one-hundred kids each summer.

Most of Dorris's residents consisted of farmers and ranchers. Larry fit right in and hit it off with the people. He also took advantage of the area's great hunting and fishing. "It turned out to be just a great place to live," he says.

Larry enjoyed the older people as much as the younger. He visited seniors regularly, and they often invited the Brownings to their homes for dinner. Larry even became friends with the "church manager" deacon, though the two butted heads a few times. Larry's experience playing in a band came in handy. The older people enjoyed it when he and a friend named Les sang duets at church potlucks.

Larry honed his preaching skills at Dorris, and typically delivered expository, verse-by-verse sermons. He gave messages intended to encourage, build up and equip believers for ministry. Although he believed, and still believes, in eternal punishment in hell for unbelievers, Larry wasn't a fire-and-brimstone preacher. He occasionally gave evangelistic sermons, especially on Easter and at Christmastime, when higher numbers of non-Christians attended.

On Sunday mornings they sang only hymns from hymnals. On Wednesdays nights, Larry played guitar and led the congregation in contemporary choruses.

In the summer of 1990, Larry came home to a surprise. Karen presented him with a wrapped little present. He opened it to find a pair of baby shoes. She just smiled. It took several seconds for Larry to catch on that Karen was pregnant. The news thrilled him.

On February 5, 1991, in a Klamath Falls, Oregon hospital, Karen entered the final stages of labor. Larry watched in awe as the doctor delivered Paige and cleaned out her mouth so she could take her first breaths.

"I was overwhelmed by the fact that she started from a seed and turned into a little baby," recalls Larry. "I wept for joy at Paige's birth."

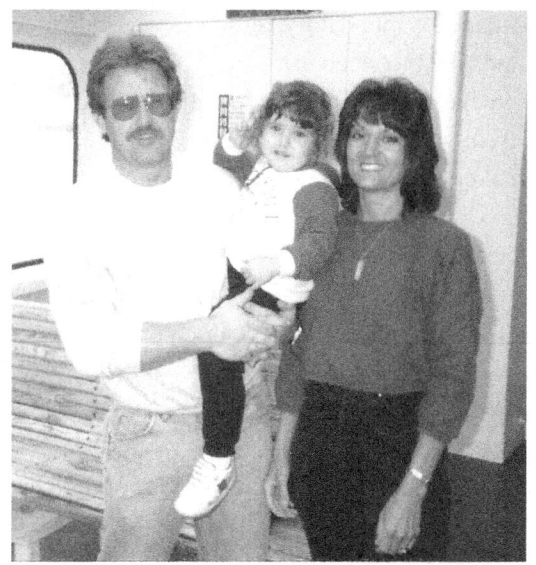

Pastor Larry, Paige and Karen. 1993 or '94.

৵৩৩

10

MINISTRY

A van pulls into the parking lot of the Eugene Mission. The wheelchair ramp unfolds, and the driver, Dick Burke, rolls Larry out and onto the pavement. It's the fourth Thursday of the month and four men from McKenzie Bible Fellowship (MBF) have arrived for ministry. They enter the building and make their way to the empty chapel. It will soon be filled with an all-male congregation. The MBF men distribute one hundred or so song sheets on the pews.

Larry will be the main speaker tonight.

The audience of mostly homeless men begins to file in.

Chapel attendance is mandatory for these "guests" if they hope for dinner and a bed to sleep in.

Each evening, chapel services are conducted by volunteers from various churches or Christian groups within Lane County. Speakers face a captive audience of primarily disinterested, resistant listeners, many of whom feign coughing and throat-clearing as a mass show of defiance. Occasional smart-mouthed remarks surface as well, although too much overt defiance won't be tolerated by the staff. So a minimum of order exists, though rebellion simmers near the surface.

It takes courage to be a chapel speaker at the Eugene Mission.

[Note: a few years later, the mission would change chapel policy, making attendance voluntary. Although the numbers decreased, attitudes improved.]

Three men lift Larry and his wheelchair onto the stage. They position him beside the pulpit. Someone places a microphone, attached to a long boom, above Larry's head.

The music leader, Barry Bryan, strums a guitar and begins to sing. The MBF men join him in a few worship songs. Only a handful of the guests participate in the singing.

The music ends and the MBF youth pastor, Dean Redding, stands at the pulpit and gives some opening comments. The loud coughing and throat-clearing begin. If one didn't know better, it would seem that most of the men have a cold, bronchitis, emphysema or worse.

Dean introduces Larry, then sits down with the other MBF men near the back wall of the stage.

Someone adjusts the boom so the microphone is near Larry's mouth. He begins. "If you have your Bibles... [breathe] ...turn to Luke nineteen. I won't... [breathe] ...be using a Bible,... [breathe] ...because I can't see. So I'm... [breathe]

...going to narrate this story... [breathe] ...for you."

The faux coughing and throat-clearing stop. The audience decides to show respect to this weak-voiced blind man in the wheelchair.

Larry tells the story of Zacchaeus, the wealthy, despised and physically short tax collector of Jericho, who climbed a sycamore tree so he could gaze over the crowd at Jesus. As Jesus passed by, he looked up in the tree and said, "Zacchaeus, make haste and come down, for today I must abide at your house."

Larry explains how Zacchaeus scrambled down the tree and joyfully promised to give half his goods to the poor and restore fourfold to everyone he'd defrauded. Jesus declared that salvation had come to Zacchaeus's house. The self-righteous crowd murmured against Jesus for intending to eat dinner at this sinner's house.

Larry makes a few more points, then concludes. "Just as Jesus was passing through Jericho, Jesus is passing this way. The question I have for you, is he calling your name? Jesus is here and he knows each of you by name. If he's calling your name, then you need to respond like Zacchaeus and make haste—and come down and surrender your life to Christ."

Dean approaches the podium and gives an altar call. Barry leads the men through another song. No one responds to the altar call. The chapel session concludes. The MBF men linger near the exit and shake hands with the attendees as they leave for the dining area.

One young man lags behind. He approaches Dean and says he wants to receive Christ as his Savior. Dean asks Larry to explain the way of salvation to the young man.

Larry obliges. He explains that we receive salvation by first acknowledging that we are sinners. Then, we must confess our sins to God and repent of them. Larry explains that Christ died on the cross for our sins and we must accept Him as our Lord and Savior.

The young man affirms that he believes this to be true. The MBF men pray with him and he receives Jesus as his Lord and Savior. Larry then states the importance of reading the Bible and fellowshipping with Christians knowledgeable of the Scriptures.

The MBF men leave the chapel with the new Christian and they join the others for supper in the dining area. Turkey casserole is the main dish. Larry passes on dinner, having eaten beforehand. He does eat dessert, though—coconut milk ice cream. Dick Burke, a retired Wycliffe missionary, sits next to Larry and feeds him. After eating, the men return to the van, load Larry in, and head home.

ഇരു

Paige's birth filled Larry with joy and a sense of awe. A problem at the church threatened to stifle the good cheer, however. A bitter situation arose in response to Larry's withdrawal of one hundred dollars from the First Baptist youth fund to help pay for a Christian music concert in Dorris. Three other local churches had also kicked in one hundred dollars each. The concert drew over one hundred young people. "One teenager gave his life to the Lord that night," says Larry, "so I felt pretty good about it."

A church member thought Larry should have sought approval before withdrawing the money from the fund. "She got some of the people of the church to agree with her, and they were talking behind my back, just causing disunity in the body."

No church policy required Larry to seek permission to use youth-fund money for youth ministry. Prior to the concert, he had also withdrawn funds to take teens on trips to San Francisco, Marriott's Great America and the Oregon coast. He'd also used youth-fund money to finance an earlier Christian concert. Nobody criticized him for that. Also, Larry did most of the work raising money for the fund. So it pricked his pride when a few people questioned his integrity on the matter.

Most of the church supported him, but a group of about eight people kept pushing the issue. He allowed the situation to eat at him.

"Instead of dealing with it like I should have, I kind of became stiff-necked and said, 'I don't need to put up with this.'"

Larry sent out resumes to other churches. Several responses came back and he decided to pursue a pastorate at North Addison Baptist Church in Spokane, Washington. Larry took a Sunday off from Dorris and traveled north with Karen. He preached a sample sermon to the Spokane congregation and talked with the pastoral search committee. The couple returned to Dorris and waited.

"About a week later we got a call from Spokane and they voted eighty to two to call us as their pastor."

Larry had yet to tell anyone from Dorris about his decision to leave. He felt it would be best to announce his resignation after first accepting the new position. When the congregation at First Baptist heard the news, many pleaded with Larry to stay, but he stuck to his decision.

"It was probably one of the most difficult things that I had done—to leave the friends and the family we had established in Dorris."

In hindsight, Larry believes he resigned rashly, due to his immaturity. He concluded he should have remained and worked through the problem instead of running away from it. "I should have just put the one hundred dollars back in the youth fund out of my own pocket," he says. "That way they wouldn't have had anything to complain about."

When the Brownings left Dorris in July of 1991, the congregation had grown from seventeen to about eighty regular attendees, with many young people attending. Not bad for a town of just a thousand. "During that five year time together, we developed some very deep relationships with people that continue even today."

Romans 8:28 applies to our mistakes. Although Larry left Dorris for the wrong reasons, God, who knows we are but clay, worked it for good and blessed Larry's new ministry in Spokane.

Of course, part of the "good" involved God making Larry face problems similar to what he'd avoided back in Dorris. One of his early sermons at North Addison contained a bit of a confession. He told the new congregation about his mistake at leaving First Baptist and how the Lord would eventually make him learn the lesson he had refused to learn while there.

"I don't think the sermon was centered around that," he says, "but it was just a confession I made to the church, that sometimes we want to get away from our problems. We think the grass is greener on the other side, only to find that the grass is greener because it's been watered. Or, as someone else said, 'The grass is greener because the manure is deeper.'"

Larry's honeymoon period at North Addison was short. God wasted little time in making him learn what he'd he avoided by leaving Dorris. The primary lesson concerned the need to face problems, not ignore them.

When he arrived in Spokane, Larry encountered a situation where, during the interim between pastors, four members had taken too much control of a children's Sunday school class and an adult women's Bible study. Initiative can be good, but they were running the classes without touching base with the new pastor. Larry didn't ask them to quit teaching the classes; he simply pressed for more accountability. The four teachers didn't respond well to the criticism and eventually quit the church.

The new pastor faced another test. He noticed that the Sunday school director never attended Sunday school, but instead spent class time walking around the church with his little boy, who also didn't attend. The director didn't even drop in on classes to check up on them.

One day, Larry asked why he didn't attend and the man simply said he didn't want to. Larry told him that as Sunday school director, he and his son needed to attend classes. The man refused and soon stopped going to church altogether.

Larry learned that you can't solve problems by wishing them away. By intervening, he kept problems from getting worse, though a few members quit.

The Brownings moved to Spokane in July of 1991. Larry was 41, Karen 34 and Paige six months old. On a typical Sunday morning, the congregation at North Addison numbered from ninety to one hundred, with a balanced mix of older folks, middle-aged, young adults and youth. Those numbers remained the same during the Brownings four years at North Addison.

Larry saw more suits and ties in the Washington church, compared to the jeans and overalls worn at his first pastorate. Other than differences in dress, the city folk of Spokane and the country folk at Dorris shared the same basic human traits. His sermons at North Addison differed little from those at the small California town. "People are still the same when it comes to spiritual things," he affirms. "The Bible says that our job is to equip the saints for the work of the ministry, so I really tried to focus on that."

Larry placed value in the Sunday sermon, but his

ministry worked best seven days a week, as he developed relationships with individuals. He loved spending time with senior adults, whether fishing for Kokanee salmon with an elderly widow or holding weekly Bible studies at retirement centers.

Larry experienced something odd in late summer of 1991. He saw a blue haze through his left eye. It was as if everything in his vision was filtered through a blue lens. The right eye's vision remained normal. He visited an ophthalmologist, who conducted several tests and found nothing wrong.

"In hindsight," says Larry, "You would have thought that an ophthalmologist would know that it's one of the signs [of MS], that if you can't find anything wrong, it's something neurological."

The bluish vision continued for about four months, then went away. Everything else in his body worked fine, and he soon forgot about the haze.

The odd visual anomaly failed to curb Larry's passion for ministry. He enjoyed youth snow camps and ski trips as much as the kids did. Vacation Bible School thrived during his stay at North Addison.

Larry often held Bible studies at Spokane's jail. "I'd just go where the prisoners were, outside playing basketball, cards or whatever. I would say, 'I'm gonna have a Bible study if any of you want to join me.' There were always at least a couple of guys; we had good conversations."

Every church has members with practical needs. One person may lack food, another shelter, or perhaps a disabled person needs a ride to church. To meet such needs, Larry implemented a Southern Baptist program called Deacon Family Ministry. North Addison had six deacons. Each was given responsibility for fifteen families. A deacon would stay in regular contact with his assigned families and make sure their needs were getting met. Once a month, Larry and the deacons met for breakfast, where they discussed their work with the families. The ministry worked well and the deacons met the responsibility with enthusiasm. And most importantly, needs were met.

"I had some of the best deacons a pastor could ever want," says Larry. "They didn't want any power or anything. All they wanted to do was serve."

The members of North Addison had built a new church just before Larry's arrival. Rather than sell the old building, they rented it to a group of Russian Christians. The Russians often invited the Brownings to their fellowship dinners; the women insisted that Larry sample large portions of each type of food. He'd leave the dinners stuffed. Saying "nyet" would have been rude.

Since the pastorate was full time, Larry didn't need to find other work. He could focus his energy on ministry. He also took on the duties of youth pastor and church secretary. Eventually the church found people for those positions.

Karen focused primarily on baby Paige. A few years later, when Paige entered preschool, Karen found a job as a teacher's aide.

Larry and Karen opened their home for anyone who wanted to drop by for fellowship—or a swim. They purchased a home that had an in-ground pool, and invited people to come anytime for a dip.

Karen taught children's Sunday school and became involved with a ministry called Team Moms that met Tuesday nights at the church. She had her hands full, caring for Paige and working as a teacher's aide.

The Lord blessed Larry's stay at North Addison even though his initial purpose was to seek greener grass. He reflects fondly of one particular accomplishment. For about three summers, Larry and a few others from North Addison traveled north to Williams Lake, British Columbia, to assist a small church with Vacation Bible School. This mission outreach from Spokane provided much energy and encouragement for the fledgling flock, which eventually grew into a large church.

On January 13, 1995, Karen underwent an early-morning surgery to deaden nerves in the back of her uterus. The procedure would relieve frequent menstrual cramps she had endured for years.

Larry and Paige waited at the hospital during the surgery. After just forty-five minutes, the surgeon emerged and announced that the operation went well.

Larry and Paige sat in the waiting area while Karen remained in recovery. After a long wait, Larry decided to check on her.

"I went to the door and looked into the recovery room," he says. "Karen was in tremendous amounts of pain."

He asked the nurse what was wrong and she wasn't sure. The surgeon had left soon after the procedure. The nurses had administered all the pain medications the doctor had ordered. The pain persisted. Meanwhile, the nurses tried in vain to contact the doctor. Larry insisted they keep trying.

The hospital had a policy where doctors did not intervene on another doctor's patient. So the only doctor who would order pain killers was the one who performed Karen's surgery. At about 5 p.m., Karen said, "Larry, go ahead and just take Paige home."

The surgeon called Larry the next morning, a Saturday, and said they would perform a CAT scan to isolate the problem. Larry told the doctor he'd be right there. He dropped Paige off at a church member's home and drove to the hospital. He waited about four hours without anyone giving him updates on his wife's condition.

Finally, the surgeon came out, accompanied by another surgeon. The doctors informed Larry that Karen's bowel had been pierced during the previous day's surgery. Toxins had leaked into her system throughout the night. The second doctor had performed corrective surgery, fixing the hole in her bowel. The two physicians said she would be fine, but Larry felt the second surgeon seemed abrasive and uncaring.

Larry visited Karen that morning, soon after they moved her from recovery. "She seemed to be feeling a whole lot better," says Larry. "So I got Paige and brought her back."

Larry and Paige stayed with Karen until about 8:30 p.m.. She sat up, talked and claimed to feel fine. The doctors suggested she'd require a seven day hospital stay. Larry felt things were under control, so he and Paige went home. He intended to go ahead with the next day's church service.

The Browning's phone rang at 2:30 a.m. Sunday. It was the doctor who had performed Karen's corrective surgery. He told Larry they were moving Karen to the intensive care unit (ICU) for better care, that there was nothing to be concerned about, and he didn't need to come immediately. Larry went back to sleep, assuming she was in good hands. Later, he would discover that her blood pressure had dropped very low and her skin had turned an ashen color. The doctor brushed it off as dehydration.

At 6:30 a.m. a nurse called. "Mr. Browning, you need to get to the hospital right now."

"What's going on?" asked Larry.

"You just need to get here right now," she answered.

He dropped Paige off at the home of an older couple from their church and rushed to the hospital. He waited.

Two doctors approached him. One of them said, "Mr. Browning, your wife has suffered a severe heart attack. The left side of her heart has quit functioning."

Larry reacted with shock and disbelief. The doctors asked for Larry's permission to perform angioplasty, widening the damaged coronary artery with a balloon catheter. Larry said yes. He then called a few members of North Addison, told them things were very serious and he wouldn't be able to conduct the service that morning. Several members arrived to offer him support.

Angioplasty proved ineffective. Karen's heart failed to improve.

Larry recalls his state of mind. "I was very angry with the doctors because of their lack of concern. I was just in a state of shock, thinking, *How could this happen in a hospital, where they're supposed to be giving you the best care?* I was just numb. I couldn't believe it."

He asked the doctor, "In your honest opinion, what are my wife's chances?"

"Mr. Browning, in my honest opinion, your wife is going to die."

Larry thought, *This happens to other people.* He wept. Distraught, he prayed that God would not let Karen die.

Larry called Karen's mother, Mary, and four sisters, Patti, Sharon, Diane and Michelle. He said they needed to get to Spokane immediately. Karen's father had passed away previously. Larry called his own family. Members of North Addison Church continued to arrive. A prayer vigil began in the waiting area.

"I went in to see Karen and they had her on a life-support system. She was really swollen from her head to her toes and didn't even look like herself. She was unresponsive."

Larry sat with her, held her hand, prayed. He left her room for a short time to pray with the people in the waiting area. The doctors tried several other procedures, but Karen failed to improve.

At around 5 p.m. that Sunday, Larry's mother, Agatha, arrived in Spokane with her husband, Lynn. They first stopped at Larry and Karen's house to visit Paige, still under the care of the older couple. The little girl, nearly four years old, met her grandmother outside. Agatha remembers Paige saying, "Grandma, my mom is dying."

Agatha, not yet aware of Karen's prognosis, said, "Oh no, honey, she's just really sick."

Early Sunday evening, Karen's sisters and mother arrived. They spent time alone with her.

"I don't think she was even alive at that time," says Larry. "They had her on life support and were feeding her with [medications] that kept her blood pressure up a little bit. So we prayed through the night."

The next morning, Monday, the doctors told Larry that kidney dialysis might help. The toxins from the pierced bowel had circulated in Karen's system for about twenty-four hours prior to the corrective surgery. Her kidneys, along with other vital organs, had been severely damaged. The dialysis began.

"She coded [went into cardiac arrest]," says Larry, "They brought her back. They tried the dialysis again, and she coded again. They brought her back."

The doctors told Larry the dialysis didn't work—that they couldn't do anything else for her.

Paige, three weeks shy of her fourth birthday, arrived with the older couple who had been watching over her.

"Dad made the decision that he didn't want me to remember her like that," recalls Paige, "so he didn't let me see her. We were in this little waiting room, and I just remember crying because I didn't know what was happening. I knew that she was sick—and he told me that I couldn't see her. It probably would have scared me more than anything. I know that was the hardest thing for him to do."

Larry met with Karen's mother and sisters. "I asked them, 'What do you think we should do?' At that point I had decided that I wanted to take her off life support, because I thought that was all that was really keeping any functions going. I didn't think Karen was still there. Karen and I had talked before and we both said that if we ever got into that position—that we did not want to be kept alive by life support.

"So her mother, sisters and I all agreed that we should take her off life support. I told the doctor that we wanted to shut off the life support."

The procedure would involve, first, a slow withdrawal of the intravenous blood pressure medications. Then they would turn off the ventilator.

Larry, Karen's sisters and mother watched as a nurse gradually shut off the medications. A respiratory therapist began to turn down the ventilator. The cardiac monitor flat-lined.

"Before they could even get the life support off, there was no brain activity, there was no heart activity. They pronounced her dead on January sixteenth at around two in the afternoon."

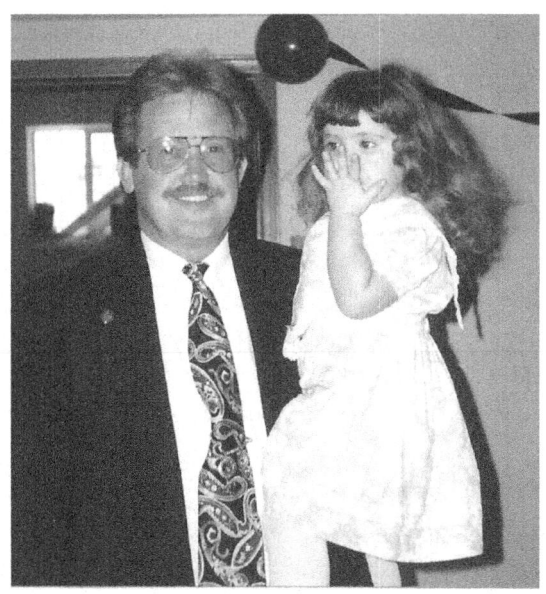

Larry and Paige, mid-1990's

৪০৫৪

11
SHADOWLANDS

Paige arrived home last night from Los Angeles, having just completed her second year of nursing school at California Baptist University in Riverside. I'm cleaning up in the kitchen and hear her footsteps descending the stairway. She enters her father's room. I hear her say, "Good morning, Dad." He's in the standing frame, so they're able to talk at the same level.

Larry's half-hour session in the standing frame is about over. I enter his room and notice Paige's right arm around him in a half hug. Their heads are touching. The equipment prevents a full embrace. They're praying. Not wanting to interrupt, I turn around and tip-toe out of the room.

Soon, their voices return to a louder, conversational tone. I reenter the bedroom, greet Paige, and slowly release the standing frame's jack, which lowers Larry back into his wheelchair. The sensitive jack releases too quickly though, and Larry lands in his wheelchair a bit hard. Klutzy me.

He's okay, and jokingly tells Paige how his caregivers abuse him. I wince ever so slightly, hoping she doesn't take him seriously. She doesn't. The three of us chat for a bit, then I ask Paige if she would like to be interviewed sometime for the book. She says yes.

While adjusting the tilt of the wheelchair, I ask Larry if I can borrow some recordings of his old sermons. He gives me the go-ahead and tells me they're in the drawer of his bed stand.

"His sermons were good," says Paige.

"I wasn't too bad of a preacher," he responds.

I open the drawer and take out three cassettes, two from early 2002, and one from August 2005 titled *Pastor Larry's Last Sermon as Pastor of Valley Hills.*

"Anything else I can help you with?" I ask.

"Nope. You have a good day, Tom," says Larry.

I say goodbye. With cassettes in hand, I leave the house and get into my pickup. The tape from January 2002, is titled *Hope When You Are Depressed: Part One (Revelation 1:1-8).* I insert the cassette into my pickup's stereo and back out of the driveway.

Larry gave this sermon about two months after his MS diagnosis. He could still walk, though his left leg dragged. His arms and vision worked fine. In the recording, Larry sounds like a different man. He speaks strong, clear, fast, with few pauses. He's articulate, tossing in fifty-cent words now and then. His knowledge of Scripture is very good. The preaching is better than I expected—the voice of a pro.

"He never preached fluffy sermons," says Ryan of his father. "His sermons had real substance…deep, but still easy to understand. He preached on the level of those he was speaking to."

Those who knew Larry prior to his MS find it difficult facing him in his advanced stages of the disease. He has mentioned disappointment that many good friends from his past have not visited. "People are busy with full schedules," he says.

And that may be true. It's also true, I think, that many of those old friends are *afraid* to see him and feel guilty about it. What should be a simple visit becomes something monumental, so they keep putting it off. All Larry wants to do is reconnect with them, maybe just shoot the breeze.

It appears that many fair-weather friends have deserted him. Though Ann is hurt by the abandonment, she is not bitter or consumed by it. She says, "I hear a lot of people say, 'I just want to remember Larry the way he was.' Well, you just don't have that privilege. That is just so selfish. It's kind of like people are either real and helpful, or else they just bail. It's like there's not a lot of in-between."

It's painful to see Larry in his current state. It's especially painful for those who knew him when he was healthy. And if they muster up the nerve to visit him, what then? Should they cry and sob over his condition? No. Larry's had enough of that. I've never seen him cry, so it seems inappropriate for others to get weepy around him. I think the next step is to look beyond the disability to the heart of the man. It's about friends reconnecting, talking, laughing, caring.

I think it's easier for me—never having seen Larry walk, run or shoot a basketball. The Larry of today is the man I know, not the strong, energetic preacher from the cassette. Having not known the healthy Larry may help me do a better job as his caregiver.

Ann, Paige, Ryan and Agatha have suffered heartbreak over each phase of Larry's decline. And their hearts continue to break. In the midst of that anguish, they continue to love him.

They have not bailed.

ഔൽ

Inside the ICU, Larry wept with Karen's mother and sisters. Just three days earlier, Karen had overflowed with health and vigor. Now she lay still, the victim of a botched surgical procedure.

Nearby, in a small room, a tearful Paige waited with the couple from church.

A few days after Karen's death, Larry took Paige to the funeral home to view her mother's body. The swelling was gone and the mortician applied makeup well. She appeared to be sleeping. Larry explained to his daughter, not yet four, that the body was just clay, and her mother was in heaven with Jesus. "I don't think Paige really understood," he says.

About 400 people attended Karen's funeral at North Addison. Several pastors from across the Northwest attended. Larry spoke during the service, sharing his confidence that Karen was with the Lord, that she loved her family and friends, and that her hope and prayer would be for those present to find Jesus as their Lord and Savior.

Paige remembers the funeral. "I felt detached from it, like I was almost watching myself. I didn't cry when I saw her. It was like I was numb."

Another service was held in Springfield, Oregon, at

Trinity Baptist, Larry's childhood church. About 300 attended. Several from Dorris, California drove up to show their support. Karen was buried at Springfield Memorial Gardens where Larry's dad had been buried.

In the days that followed, Larry grieved mostly alone with God. Sometimes, while Paige was being cared for at a church member's home, Larry would weep and pray, "God, why? Why did this have to happen?"

When people asked how he was doing, he'd answer, "I'm doing fine," which is how he responds to this day. One could argue he was/is being dishonest, but the straight answer would be anguishing, exhausting, and involve more than the questioner really intended.

In the aftermath of Karen's death, Larry and Paige were nearly inseparable. As he settled back into his pastoral duties, he enrolled her in a preschool, conveniently located in the church. Paige enjoyed being around other kids.

Though he questioned God during this period of brokenness and grief, Larry didn't turn from Him. The Lord used the intense trial to refine Larry's character and make him a better man. "One of the deacons told me that my ministry had become more effective in that time since Karen died. He said I was able to relate to more people. I think he was referring to my sermons, my attitude and actions."

In the spring of 1995, three or four months after Karen's death, Larry took a week off to seek God's direction. Agatha stayed with Paige while he took a trip to Alaska. Along with prayer and soul-searching, he enjoyed some fishing.

That same year, a friend recommended that Larry file suit against the doctor who pierced Karen's bowel, as well as the doctor who repaired the bowel. Larry contacted a law firm. The lawyers thought there was strong evidence to pursue two separate suits against the doctors. On their advice, Larry settled out of court and received $200,000 from the doctor who pierced the bowel. After lawyers fees and other expenses, Larry kept about $134,000. Looking back, he believes his lawyers gave him bad advice to settle with the first doctor. Larry feels if it had gone to trial, he probably would have won the suit and received substantially more money.

In the second suit, the surgeon who repaired the bowel refused to settle and it took four years before it came to trial. Larry believed the surgeon had procrastinated before performing the corrective surgery. The delay allowed toxins to continue leaking into Karen's system. Larry felt the surgeon was rude and resisted involvement with Karen's care. He was found guilty of negligence, but not to the point of her death, so Larry received no money from the second suit.

"I know that I prayed and asked for God's leadership. I really believe that if I had received a large amount of money, I would have been less dependent on God in the future. Therefore, perhaps it was God's will that I didn't win."

In May of 1995, Larry's sister Brenda, a school nurse, called from Springfield. She gave him the phone number of a single brunette named Ann, a florist and dress designer. She had a nine-year-old son, Ryan.

Not one to be shy, Larry gave Ann a call. They hit it off and, for the next few weeks, talked by phone for two hours nearly every night. Larry caught a flight to Eugene and met Ann in person on May 24. Their first date included dinner at a popular Mexican restaurant, followed by a movie. Then he flew back to Spokane.

At the end of July, Larry announced his resignation to the North Addison congregation. "I thought it was best for us to move back to Springfield where I had family [his mother and sister], and they could help me take care of Paige. Another reason was so that I could be close to where Ann lived and build our relationship."

He pastored at North Addison for another month before moving to Springfield, where he found a truck-driving job.

Larry received some criticism for dating only six months after Karen's death. His grief continued even while he saw Ann. He saw the reality of his situation. "After being married seventeen years, I didn't really look forward to being alone, and I had a four year old daughter who needed a mother."

In the months after he resigned from North Addison, Larry traveled much with Paige to places such as the Grand Canyon and Yellowstone. They also spent a month in Tennessee and North Carolina where Paige connected with her relatives for the first time. She celebrated her fifth birthday with Larry's cousins in North Carolina.

Back home in Springfield, Oregon, Larry grew closer to Ann and her son, Ryan. "I had come to care deeply about Ann and Ryan, and I thought that she would make a wonderful mother for Paige."

Ann doesn't remember when Larry first popped the big question. "I don't think there was a specific proposal. He just really wanted to get married, from right when we first started dating. He just kept relentlessly asking and asking and asking."

Eventually Ann said yes. Practical thinking played a significant role in her decision. "He was positive, active, fun-loving, loved the Lord. I really think the kids had a lot to do with it too, because Ryan wanted a dad so bad, and Paige wanted a mom. When you've been hurt the way I was [in her previous marriage], you're not, like, all crazy in love. It's just not like that. At least it wasn't for me."

Says Ryan about the marriage: "I liked the idea—I think

because it made me feel like we had a normal family and not a broken one."

Larry and Ann married on May 31st, 1996 at Ann's church, Grace Community Fellowship. Her pastor conducted the ceremony. Ann wore a creamy white satin gown with lace around the top and back.

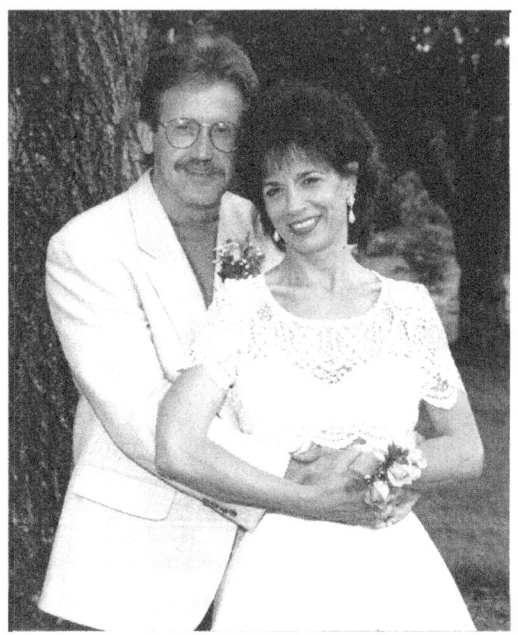

Ann and Larry, wedding day, May 31, 1996

Larry wore a sport jacket, a nice t-shirt and a pair of jeans. The combination worked well, and it's worth noting that actor Don Johnson popularized the look in the trendsetting 1980's cop show, Miami Vice. Though Larry's jacket wasn't a thousand-dollar Versace, it still looked pretty snazzy.

Did Ann approve of his casual look? "It was my idea," she says. "I don't like guys in slacks. I like jeans."

Ann and Larry honeymooned in Sedona, Arizona for a week, then returned to Springfield. They moved into her house on South 70th Street.

Life as a blended family began. "I don't think it was as hard for us to blend in as for some," says Larry, "namely because we had Christ at the center of our lives."

Says Ann, "The worst annoying thing was that Paige and Ryan argued all the time. Having just one kid, you don't have that. It was just for attention. They wanted Larry's attention more than mine. When he was gone, they were fine."

As a single dad, Larry had too often resorted to fast food for meals. With Ann, that all changed. Says Paige, "Dad fed me junk food, and Ann, Mom, cooked good food for us."

The family decided to attend Ann's church, Grace Community Fellowship. Paige initially resisted the switch from Trinity, where her grandparents attended. She also had to adjust to sharing her dad with a new mom and brother.

Likewise, Ryan had to adjust. "I didn't like the idea of having a little sister. All my life I had been an only child; I liked playing by myself."

Ann did most of the counseling with the children and helped them work through emotional issues. Says Larry, "I'd just go have fun with the kids. She'd have to deal with all their frustrations."

Larry found employment at Kintigh's Mountain Home Ranch, a Christmas tree farm owned by Ann's family. He worked there for about a year and a half, earning the respect of his new in-laws.

God's calling still burned in Larry's heart and he hoped to return to full-time ministry. Soon after he and Ann married, Larry voiced his desire that the family move to northern Italy as missionaries. He'd learned about a mission opportunity near a

U.S. Air Force base in Aviano.

Ann felt that such a drastic change so soon could have a detrimental effect on the children, who were still recovering from past traumas. Says Ann, "What I absolutely did not want to do was to move somewhere far away, because Ryan and Paige were both so traumatized."

Larry and Ann agreed to hold off on big changes for a year. But at the same time, Larry was primed to do anything for Jesus.

Ann recalls him often saying, "I don't care—I'll go live in a tent. If it's God's will that I live in a tent, then I'll live in a tent."

Says Ann, "And you know, he probably would have lived in a tent. We talked about that later on [when he was in advanced stages of MS] and I said, 'This is way worse than living in a tent.'"

During the first year of marriage, Larry filled in as an interim pastor at two churches. He regularly preached at a Baptist church in the town of Veneta. The congregation wanted him to stay as a permanent, part-time pastor. Larry declined. He wanted a full-time pastorate and Veneta was a long commute from Springfield.

Larry also filled in at a non-denominational church in east Springfield, close to home. The congregation wanted Larry to preach regularly while they searched for a full-time minister. He agreed to preach occasionally, but a problem arose because of the church's doctrinal statement. It stated that a believer could lose their salvation under some circumstances. Larry, a Calvinist and staunch believer in the eternal security of Christians, respectfully told them, "…unless you denounce the doctrine, I can't preach [regularly]."

The church didn't change their doctrinal statement, but

they were happy to have Larry preach whenever he could. Eventually, they hired a permanent minister. Larry continued to seek God's direction.

In June of 1997, he filled out a survey and sent it to the headquarters of the Southern Baptist Convention. The survey assessed his skills and determined his suitability for planting a new church.

The results of the survey indicated that Larry possessed the aptitude and strengths needed for starting a church from scratch. He met with two Southern Baptist organizers: the New Work Start Strategist and the Associational Missionary, who offered him encouragement and counsel. Larry arrived at a decision: he would plant a new church.

The Southern Baptist Convention and its Missions Association agreed to support him in a "phase-in program" where he would receive funding for three years upon planting the church. The program required that he meet specific goals during each phase of the startup. If he failed to meet the goals, the funding would be cut off.

In the summer of 1997, Larry again saw a blue haze in the vision of his left eye. Ann encouraged him to see an ophthalmologist. Larry resisted, telling her, "Well, if I go to an ophthalmologist, it's going to cost me a hundred dollars and he's going to tell me he doesn't know what's wrong."

Ann insisted, so he made an appointment. As Larry predicted, the eye doctor failed to diagnose the cause of the blue haze—and charged about one hundred dollars. As in 1991, the haze went away after about four months. The rest of his body functioned well and he continued planning the startup.

Larry prepared a video and a pamphlet describing the new work. He mailed several copies to friends, family and various churches. A core group of about fifteen people formed, committing themselves to planting the church. Larry named it Valley Hills Community Church because of the many hills surrounding east Springfield. "And rather than call it Valley Hills *Baptist,* we felt we could reach more people by…the *community* approach."

The core group met weekly in the Browning home to pray, study the Bible and seek God's direction on how to reach out to the community.

Larry used ideas from Rick Warren's book *The Purpose-Driven Church* (Zondervan, 1995), which emphasizes a church's health over growth. Five biblical purposes are outlined in the book: "Love the Lord with all your heart," "Love your neighbor as yourself," "Go and make disciples," "Baptize them," and "Teach them to obey."

Larry conducted a survey in the community asking people why they didn't go to church. When he analyzed the results, one reason topped the list: people thought the church was just after their money. Second, they believed sermons were boring and lacked life application. Third, churches were too formal in areas such as dress.

After several months of planning, Larry and the core group set a launch date of April 12, 1998—Easter Sunday. "It was also my dad's birthday," says Larry.

They mailed out 7,000 fliers throughout east Springfield, inviting people to attend Valley Hills' first service at the Thurston High School auditorium. Larry and Ann had both graduated from Thurston. Ann would decorate and handle preparation of a continental breakfast for the attendees.

The week before Easter, they conducted a trial run in the Thurston auditorium and about 100 people showed up, wrongly expecting a continental breakfast. They had misread the flier, which said the breakfast would be on Easter. The trial run was well worth it, though, because bugs needed working out, such as a faulty sound system.

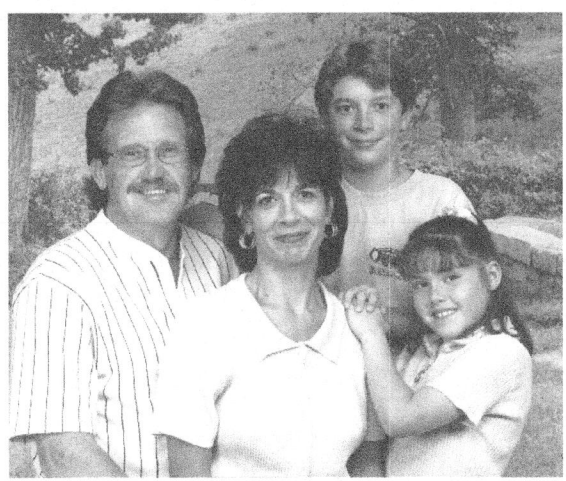

Family photo, 1998. Larry, Ann, Ryan and Paige.

The opening day, on Easter, went well. The sound system worked fine and Larry delivered a message titled *Why is Easter so Important?* 265 people attended and were rewarded with the breakfast Ann prepared.

A tragedy occurred at Thurston High School in the morning of May 21, 1998, when fifteen year old Kip Kinkel arrived on campus wearing a trench coat concealing a semi-automatic rifle and two pistols. He shot two students in a hallway. Then he entered the cafeteria, where he opened fire on several others. A wounded student bravely took a second bullet while tackling Kinkel. Other students helped subdue and pin Kinkel to the floor until police arrived.

Two students died and twenty-five were wounded in the attack. It was later discovered that Kinkel had murdered his parents at their home the day before.

Valley Hills Community Church had been conducting services at Thurston for only six weeks. The Sunday after the shootings, the campus entrance was still blocked by cordons. National news vans and trucks parked along the street, just outside the school's main gate.

Instead of canceling church, Larry held a memorial service for the deceased and wounded students at a park across the street from the school. News crews filmed the memorial and segments were aired nationwide. During the service, the church took a love offering and raised $800 for the families affected by the shootings.

Valley Hills continued to meet at Thurston for the next two years. Weekly attendance ranged between 120-130 people. The auditorium held up to five-hundred. In 2000, the congregation moved to nearby Ridgeview Elementary School.

The members at Valley Hills were young, mostly in their early thirties. From the outset, Larry decided the church would be contemporary in its orientation, with trendy music and casual dress.

Each Sunday, volunteers set up and took down chairs. Larry felt that renting inhibited church growth. It was a bit of predicament, because in order to afford a building, membership needed to grow, but the growth would remain stunted until the congregation owned a building. "People get tired of having to do all the work," says Larry.

Visitors who preferred anonymity probably felt exposed at Valley Hills. Larry actively promoted fellowship. At the end of each service, he hustled to the exit to chat with people before they left the building. To stimulate relationships, coffee and refreshments were always provided afterwards.

Once a month, Ann and Larry hosted coffee and snacks at their home so new people could learn about the church. They continued the continental breakfast each Easter. The church formed a city league softball team, which Larry played on. At Valley Hills, no one sat unnoticed.

Larry emphasized commitment within the body of Christ, both in a global sense (missions) and a local sense (one's neighborhood fellowship). He chose the name Valley Hills *Community* Church for a reason. Larry encouraged official membership and offered a class for that purpose. An individual's membership would lapse unless renewed every year. "We did that so we'd know who we could count on," he says. Valley Hills was not for the commitment-phobic.

Under Larry's leadership, Valley Hills became a multifaceted hub of ministry. Each year, the men attended Promise Keepers meetings. Children looked forward to Vacation Bible School every summer. The church hosted an annual Christmas dinner at the Leaburg Community Center and invited the public. Larry regularly performed the duties expected of a pastor, such as visiting the sick and the elderly.

Through all the busyness of pastoring a fledgling church, Larry balanced well his responsibilities as a father and husband. He coached Ryan's Kidsports baseball team one season. Each month, he took Paige and Ryan out on date nights or date days, where they could do whatever they wanted. Paige would have her date with her dad on a separate day from Ryan's date, so each child received full attention from Larry.

Says Ryan of the dates, "We mostly did things that involved the outdoors—fishing, shooting, etc. I also remember going to events like car shows."

Larry helped chaperone Ryan's eighth grade class on an eight-day trip to Washington D.C., Philadelphia, Boston and New York. "We went to Gettysburg, Amish country, D.C. and all the memorials," says Larry. "I saw the Vietnam Memorial. We did all kinds of things; there's so much history back there."

In March 1999, the Brownings moved to their current home in the picturesque McKenzie River valley. Larry owned a drift boat and regularly took new people from the church on fishing trips down the river.

Ann contributed greatly to the startup and ministry of Valley Hills. She regularly employed her gift of hospitality during church-related events at their home. Ann, a professional florist, held flower potting parties (dinner included) each spring for the women at the church.

The transition to being a pastor's wife challenged Ann. "It's real lonely, I think because I was used to a home group [from her previous church] with a lot of couples my age and a lot of friends. I really had to force myself to get into the servant mode."

One day in the spring of 2001, Larry and Ann took a relaxing stroll along a canal that flows near the base of the foothills of the McKenzie valley. After several minutes, Larry noticed that his left leg dragged intermittently. He figured the problem was a pinched nerve.

That summer, while pitching on his church-league softball team, he repeatedly lost balance when he moved backwards. Then, at bat, when he'd hit the ball and run the bases, he'd stumble, sometimes falling.

Larry went on a four mile hike to a high mountain lake with Ryan and another teenager, Steve Neet. Ryan recalls how gutsy his father was on the trip: "It's one of my favorite memories of all time. I remember him getting frustrated because he couldn't walk as well as he could before. In spite of that, he carried the heaviest pack. He was a very tough man."

As the summer of 2001 ended, Larry experienced burning sensations in his right leg. The pain began in his foot and moved to the knee. Again, he assumed it was a pinched nerve.

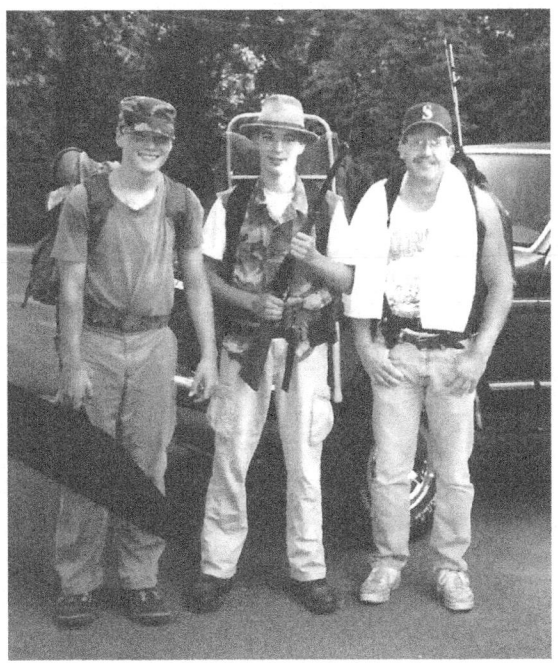

Ryan (middle) with friend and Larry. Duffy Lake, 2001.

Each fall, Larry earned supplemental income at Kintigh's Mountain Home Ranch, the Christmas tree farm owned by Ann's family. He hauled multiple armloads of fir tree seedlings out of greenhouses and loaded them into trucks. The work involved a great deal of walking back and forth. In the autumn of 2001, his left leg dragged so badly that he needed Paige, ten, and Ryan, fourteen, to help him with the hauling.

In September, he had an appointment with his doctor and they talked mostly about the painful heat sensation in his leg. The doctor took x-rays and had an MRI (magnetic resonance imaging) done on Larry's brain. They scheduled another appointment to discuss the results. During the wait, Larry visited a chiropractor two or three times, without benefit.

Larry and Ann then met with the doctor as scheduled. He told them that the x-rays and the MRI showed nothing unusual. The doctor recommended that Larry see a neurologist.

He visited a neurologist, who conducted several tests. Larry mentioned the two instances, in 1991 and 1997, when the vision in his left eye turned hazy blue. The neurologist performed a VEP (Visually Evoked Potential) test, where Larry viewed black and white checkered patterns on a TV screen. The exam revealed slow visual responses in his eyes, indicating problems with his optic nerves. Next, the neurologist took another MRI of Larry's brain, with negative results. But an MRI of Larry's spinal cord showed some irregularity near the top.

Then came a lumbar puncture, commonly know as a spinal tap. Larry heard stories of splitting headaches following the procedure, which involves sticking a needle between vertebrae into the spinal canal and removing fluid with a syringe. He steeled himself for the worse.

Ann accompanied him and stood by his side during the procedure. He clasped her hand as the needle penetrated his spine. "And he about broke my hand squeezing it," she recalls.

"It really didn't hurt," says Larry. "Just the thought of what he was doing made me about pass out."

A few days later, in November of 2001, Larry and Ann met with the neurologist. He didn't mince words.

"Mr. Browning, I've got bad news for you. I'm ninety-nine percent sure you have multiple sclerosis."

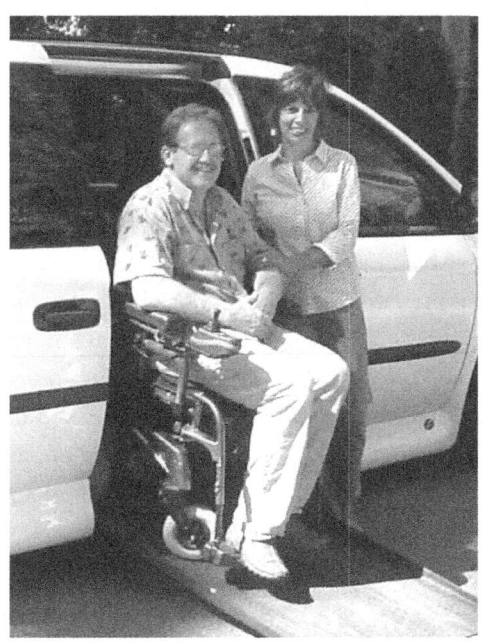

Larry and Ann. August 2004

৵৹ও

12
EVERYDAY GUY

"What people have hurt you the most in life?"

Larry and I have just discussed the ambush in Vietnam, where four of his buddies died and eight were wounded. So when I ask who's hurt him the most, I expect him to place the colonel from Vietnam at the top of the list, or perhaps the two doctors whose negligence caused Karen's death.

Instead he mentions an old girlfriend who ditched him for another guy. Then he changes his mind. Good, because it seems to me that there are far bigger hurts in life than being jilted by a girlfriend.

I brace for the deep, weighty hurt.

"Actually," he says, "I think the first person was the coach of the varsity basketball team when I tried out for basketball. I beat everybody on the team. I beat them when we were running. I beat them when we were playing one on two. Then he called me into his office and tried to get me to compare myself to the other guys on the team. When I wouldn't do it, he said, 'Well, you know, I'm going to have to cut you.' That really hurt, because I felt like I shouldn't have to be asked those questions. He saw me play, he saw what I could do, and he knew the answer."

Larry believes the coach had already chosen the team before tryouts began. Established players held a significant advantage; the coach wasn't about to pick an unknown kid from North Carolina.

Larry's story makes me wince, not at him, but at my own painful athletic history. In high school, I played on the junior varsity basketball team. Early in the season, when the coach announced the starting five, he didn't call my name. The news hurt me so badly that I gushed tears while driving home afterward.

Larry and I had developed serious hoop dreams. We both showed promise at basketball during our middle-school years, so our failures in high school marked the death of those dreams. It's a loss many athletes can relate to.

Whether it's broken hoop dreams, or singing lead vocals in a rock band, Larry's varied past enables him to relate to just about everybody. If you hang out with him for a while and look beyond his quadriplegia and blindness—it becomes clear he's an everyday guy. Good old boys share his passion for fishing, hunting, and shootin' the breeze. As a former long-haired hippie, Larry understands those on the alternative fringes. Thanks to his extensive prison ministry and druggie past, he has a heart for those trapped in crime and substance abuse. He holds a special place in his heart for elderly folks, not to mention a passion for youth ministry. In his present struggle with MS, Larry empathizes closely with those who suffer.

He can honestly say with the Apostle Paul, "I have become all things to all people, that by all means I might save some." (1 Corinthians 9:22 ESV)

Says Ryan about his father, "He spent a lot of time talking to people who would not fit in at most churches. He showed them love and friendship. There were quite a number of people at Valley Hills that came to Christ because of this."

Larry's failure to make the varsity team may bond him with others who've felt unfairly rejected, but missing the cut can hardly be considered tragic. I'm surprised that he views the coach as having hurt him so deeply.

Larry mentions other hurtful people from his past, such as the girlfriend who left him for another guy. That's a stab many have felt. Years later, when he was a pastor, a significant member of his congregation, an assumed close friend, betrayed him for no clear reason.

Certainly these are painful things, but I'm a bit perplexed. I ask him why he didn't mention the colonel in Vietnam or the doctors whose negligence caused Karen's death.

Larry acts embarrassed. "Oh, yeah, I can't believe I didn't think about those."

Perhaps some memories are too horrible to be labeled simply as hurts. They are the unmentionables that tend to be stuffed inside.

৪০৫৪

When the neurologist diagnosed him, Larry failed to understand the gravity of the situation. He knew little about MS at the time. Ann reacted more strongly, having known a wheelchair-bound uncle with MS.

Larry and Ann listened as the neurologist continued. "There are two things against you. Number one, you're a male. Number two, because of your age, it's highly likely that you have the most aggressive form of MS."

He explained that men in their early fifties, such as Larry, who develop MS, tend to get the primary-progressive (PPMS) form of the disease. Those under fifty are likely to get the relapsing-remitting (RRMS) form.

Ann felt overwhelmed by all the information, verbal and written, they received in the meeting. One piece of literature mentioned the incredible stress MS puts on marriage and how couples burdened with the disease are highly likely to divorce. After they read that, Larry, an optimist, said, "Well, I don't see why it's going to affect marriage that much."

However, Ann saw the grave reality of the situation. The healthy spouses are likely to buckle, shedding the burden of caretaking through separation or divorce. The disabled spouse can't escape, regardless of marital status. (Fast forward: over the next ten years, Ann would bear an incredible burden, but she never considered divorce. And she remained loyal to the very end.)

When the meeting with the neurologist ended, Larry failed to acknowledge the full implications of his condition. "I denied that it was going to get bad. I wasn't denying that I had MS, but when the doctor told me that it was real progressive, I kind of shrugged it off."

At home, they broke the news to Ryan, fourteen, and Paige, ten. Ryan recalls the meeting: "At the time, I wasn't very concerned because he didn't seem that bad, and I didn't really understand MS at that time." The gravity of his father's illness deeply struck Ryan a few years later, after Larry became wheelchair-bound. "When he started having trouble with other things besides his legs…it really hit me."

Paige remembers, "I just sat on the floor and cried. I think I was just scared. I didn't know what MS was, but I think it was just the fact that my dad had an incurable disease. My parents said, 'You know, we're all really scared and this is hard for us, but we're gonna get through it, because we have our faith and God will provide for us. We're not going to do this without Christ.' They just let me cry, hugged me."

Larry took a *que sera, sera* attitude and chose not to spend much time educating himself about the disease. He learned only enough to comply with whatever treatment the doctors prescribed.

The first neurologist recommended an aggressive approach and sent Larry to a cancer center for chemotherapy. Though MS is not cancer, both diseases may derive benefit from the treatment. The drugs were administered intravenously in a single session that lasted about an hour. The chemo proved ineffective in slowing the progression.

Soon after, Larry connected with a young neurologist at the Portland VA, who prescribed weekly injections of Avonex, a drug known to decrease MS flare-ups, slow progression and reduce brain lesions. The MS symptoms got worse, so the doctor ordered six more sessions of chemotherapy. That didn't work. They tried steroids, with no results. The neurologist again prescribed Avonex, which Larry injected in his thighs once a week for three years.

At this time, the VA began paying for Larry's meds and doctor visits. The Brownings had paid co-pays of $15 for each prescription and $50 for each doctor visit.

In addition to taking drugs to slow the progression of MS, Larry began taking several other meds to alleviate symptoms, such as burning pain, involuntary muscle contraction and tremors. The symptom-easing drugs worked and still work.

Through all this, Larry continued to pastor full-time at Valley Hills. "Eventually, I had to start using a cane. They had this large stool for me to sit on and people kept telling me, 'Pastor, you need to sit down.' I told them, 'When I'm ready to sit down, I'll sit down, but I'm going to stand as long as I can.'"

The relentless disease soon won and Larry finally sat on the stool to preach. During sermons, while sitting, his right leg sometimes stiffened and extended straight out. Painful cramps wrenched his thigh muscles. He would pause to explain the symptoms to the congregation.

In 2002, Valley Hills suffered a significant setback. The church's doctrinal statement listed tithing as a biblical way to give. Although tithing wasn't a requirement for membership, Larry sometimes promoted the practice in his sermons. This ruffled a particular member's feathers enough that he convinced nearly forty people to leave the church over the issue. The mass exodus disheartened Larry, but his belief in tithing remained steadfast.

By the end of 2002, he was using an electric wheelchair. He could still walk short distances if he had something to hold on to.

In 2003, Larry began using hand controls to drive the wheelchair van. He steered with the left hand and operated the throttle and brakes with his right. "You pulled it down and it would accelerate," he explains. "You pushed it forward and it would brake."

During 2004, Larry continued to prepare and deliver sermons as usual. He wrote the Sunday bulletin and performed clerical duties as he'd done since the start of Valley Hills. He could no longer walk at all. His hands and arms worked adequately. Typing became enough of a challenge that he had a voice-activated word processor installed on his computer.

Larry still drove using hand controls, but few homes had wheelchair access. So he visited church members less often. He could still maintain regular hospital visits.

At this time he began to wonder how much longer he should pastor.

The ups and downs of running a church continued. Larry typically gave Sunday school teachers a good deal of leeway and allowed them to choose their lesson plans without checking with him. In 2004, he discovered that a teacher was promoting a very rigid view of divorce to the teenage class. According to the teacher, divorce and remarriage were forbidden by God under any circumstances, even if the offending spouse committed adultery. This caused confusion for many of those teens in the class whose parents had divorced and remarried.

Valley Hills' position was less strict, stating that in a few particular instances, the Bible allowed for divorce and remarriage. Larry disliked confrontation, but felt it was needed in this situation. He said to the teacher, "It's okay for you to believe that, but it's not okay for you to teach the kids that, because it's not what the church believes or practices. If you felt so strongly about divorce being a sin, how come you never confronted Ann or me, and how could you sit under the preaching of somebody that you believed was living in sin?"

According to Christ's teaching in Matthew 19:9, it was permissible for Larry to marry Ann, a divorcee.

Larry asked the teacher to show him an outline of lessons from then on. The teacher, who had done a great job in the past, complied and continued to be involved at Valley Hills.

"I learned that I needed to be more hands-on than I was," says Larry. "I probably could have avoided a lot of conflict that went on in the church if I'd been more hands-on and not give people such a free reign. You live and learn."

The grave reality of her dad's illness hit Paige hardest at this time. The unfairness of losing her mother, and knowing she'd eventually lose her dad, caused the teenager to question her faith. "He was getting worse and he was getting worse fast. I was just really angry, even to the point I didn't want to have anything to do with God anymore. Having a mom die…and my dad, I was just brokenhearted about my dad. I can't even describe how hard it is, how hard it was."

This, along with other struggles related to being a teenager, brought Paige to a point of despair. Then, a realization hit her. She thought to herself, "Paige, you have two options. You can leave God and try to do it on your own, but you know you're not going to survive it; you're not going to be able to do this on your own. Or, you can keep going with God and just trust in Him."

She chose God. "It was because of the realization of how bad this thing was going that I recommitted my life to God." This happened at the end of her eighth-grade year.

In September 2004, Larry drove into town to visit someone at a hospital. While rounding a corner, he glanced down for a moment and reached for something, possibly a water bottle. When he looked up, cars were stopped dead in front of him. He swerved right to avoid a crash and clipped the side of a car. His van ran into the ditch.

No one at the scene claimed to be hurt. The wheelchair

van underwent much more damage than the other vehicles. Ann, at home, received a phone call from someone notifying her about the accident. She told Paige, who reacted in shock. Ann reassured her, "He's okay, he's fine. He's not hurt."

The van was totaled and the replacement didn't arrive for a few months. Larry was stuck at home.

"He was pretty crabby," says Ann.

While they waited for the new van, Larry insisted he could still drive safely using the hand controls. "That was a long, hard battle," recalls Ann. "We were all telling him not to drive, and he...this man is stubborn." Larry eventually relented and gave up the keys. From then on, he needed a driver whenever he left home. That task typically fell on Ann.

Much of Larry's ministry involved regular one-on-one fellowship, which required frequent travel to various homes. He continued to prepare and deliver sermons, but his house and hospital visits decreased significantly. Larry felt it was wrong to accept a full-time salary for part-time work.

He shared his concerns with Ann. She listened and supported him as he worked through the difficult decision. Throughout the summer of 2005, he leaned more and more toward retirement.

"It was hard to give up," says Larry, "because it was not only giving up something that I loved to do, but also it was just a reminder of my MS progressing."

He talked with the regional Southern Baptist Associational Missionary, Bill Phillips. A Springfield resident, Bill had provided strategic support during the founding of Valley Hills and became one of its first members. He also functioned as a pastor's pastor. Bill was a good sounding board and confidant. "He knew it was probably time," says Larry, "but he hated to see that day come when I had to [retire]."

The final decision rested with Larry.

Near the conclusion of a Sunday sermon, August 7, 2005, Larry announced to the congregation that he planned to retire at the end of the month.

Paige listened with tears. "I just remember that it was one of the hardest things I've ever had to hear. The thing that broke my heart the most was that he was giving up what God had called him to do. I know for him that was the hardest thing he's ever had to do."

Ann recalls, "I just remember crying. Ryan put his arms around me. Everybody was really sad. I mean, they all really loved him. It was hard. Everybody was crying."

Many in the congregation encouraged Larry to stay. They were okay with him just preaching. But he stuck to his decision. "I felt for what I was getting paid, I needed to be able to do more than that. They needed a full-time pastor."

Larry gave his final sermon as pastor of Valley Hills Community Church on August 28, 2005. It was recorded on an audio cassette. His message lacked the feel-good sentimentality one might expect in a farewell message. He used Philippians 2 as the text and challenged the congregation to shine as lights, to be blameless and hold forth the word of life. "When I stand before God," he said to them, "I will give an account of my work at Valley Hills. Whether it was in vain or not will be the proof of your lives—if you continue to live in obedience and harmony, if you continue to put feet to your faith and shine as the lights God called you to. You and I are under obligation to carry God's word to a lost and dying world."

Larry exhorted them to be transformed, renewed, and to become like Jesus so they could be examples to the lost. He challenged them to defend the faith, give to ministries, proclaim Jesus as the only way, rebuke sin, and promote holiness. His final message was tough, urging the listeners to obey God and do good works.

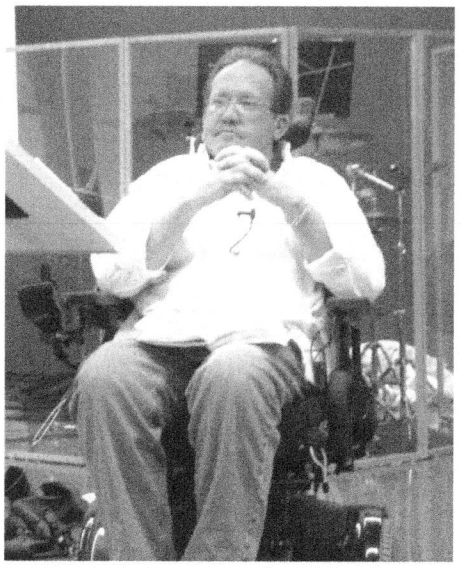

Delivering his final sermon as pastor
at Valley Hills. August 28, 2005.

Then he said goodbye. "God bless you and I thank you for the privilege of having been your pastor for this last seven and a half years. You have been a blessing to my life and to my family. I love you. I hope all of you know that I love you as my brothers and sisters in Christ—that I'm not one above you, but that I'm one of you.

"I want to encourage you that when the new pastor comes, to remember that he is the pastor and not me. If you call me pastor, I won't answer. I'll just say, 'Who are you talking to? He's not here.'

"It's been a wonderful adventure, a trying adventure. But God has been faithful—and his faithfulness has resulted in the lives of those of you that are here. I love you. God bless you. Would you pray with me?"

With those words, Larry's full-time ministry ended. His full-time tribulation began.

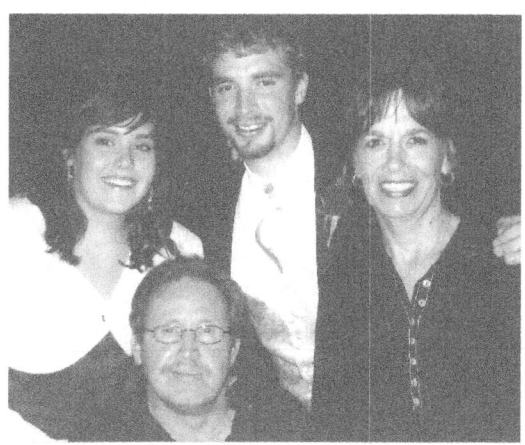

Paige, Ryan, Ann and Larry. Christmas Eve 2006

ഒരു

13
GREAT IS OUR GOD

Denise and I arrive to church late. We tiptoe into the sanctuary through a side entrance and find seats near the back. Worship music fills the air.

I'm a little edgy this morning, having stayed up late, reading apologetics defending the assertion that God is fully justified in condemning unbelievers to eternal hell. The thought of someone suffering forever in hell disturbs me, and the information helped quiet some of my anxiety on the topic. I believe hell is waiting for those who haven't placed their faith in Christ, but I still don't have a satisfactory answer to the question: "How could a loving God condemn unbelievers to an everlasting torment?"

Larry doesn't need rational justifications for hell. He

firmly believes the biblical depiction of Hades as a "place of torment" (Luke 16:28, ESV), where non-Christians will suffer for eternity. He feels badly that countless people will agonize forever, but in his view, this harsh reality should motivate Christians to work harder at sharing the gospel.

Larry was not a fire-and-brimstone preacher; his sermons were usually topical, covering a variety of issues. He says if he preached regularly today, he'd give more verse-by-verse lessons, spending several weeks on a single book of the Bible before moving on to the next. "I always presented the Gospel in my preaching," he says, "even in topical sermons. It was always focused on Jesus Christ as the answer."

As with Larry, I accept the reality of hell because the Bible says it's true. Scripture trumps my limited, human-based sense of justice. God is sovereign in how He runs His creation, and His way is perfect.

I glance at Ann and Larry, seated as usual in the left front row. My first inclination is to liken Larry's earthly existence to hell.

But no, there's a big difference. Hell involves not only punishment, but separation from God. Larry lives in close fellowship with the Lord. The future hope of actually seeing God and dwelling with Him eternally helps Larry endure the extreme hardship of quadriplegia.

I find it difficult to get into worship this morning. The choir leads the congregation through the song *How Great is Our God.* I sing along. After a few lines, I glance again at the Brownings.

Ann stands and raises her arms skyward. All others in the church remain seated. A few seconds pass and someone else stands, raising their hands. Then another. Soon, most people in the sanctuary are standing and singing.

I'm struck by the irony. Many in Ann's position would bitterly question the goodness of God. But she is the first to stand and praise Him for His greatness.

ೲೲ

Larry retired on September 1, 2005 at age fifty-five. Since his days in Dorris, he'd regularly paid into a Southern Baptist retirement account. The Southern Baptists matched his contributions. Larry would receive $458 a month, a helpful amount—but hardly enough to live on. Also, the payments wouldn't kick in for six months.

Ann now worked as Larry's caregiver 24/7. He could operate the electric wheelchair controls and feed himself with effort, but someone always needed to be available to check on him.

Says Paige of Ann, "She worked from home and had her sewing business, but I don't think that was a really big source of income. She was taking care of him now, so obviously she couldn't go out and get a job."

With very little money coming in, Larry headed straight to the Social Security office and applied for disability benefits. They accepted his application, but like the Southern Baptist pension, payments wouldn't begin for six months. So, for half a year, the Brownings would have a trickle of an income, and no savings to tide them over. They needed a miracle.

When asked how they survived for that six months, Ann gives a one-word answer: "God."

The Brownings did not ask anyone for money. They decided to trust God—and He began to work through people to supply their need. Checks started arriving in the mail. Larry's old buddy from his pre- and post-Vietnam years, Steve Keller, gave about $100 a month. A couple from the Dorris, California church pitched in. Larry's mother and stepfather gave. McKenzie Bible Fellowship, the church the Brownings would join three years later, gave them a $200 Safeway gift card. Others pitched in $100 to $150 a month. The Lord provided.

Veterans Affairs had been paying for Larry's MS medical expenses since 2001. The Brownings paid the VA co-pays of $15 for each prescription and $50 for each doctor visit.

Larry continued to seek opportunities for voluntary ministry. In 2006, he taught a Wednesday night Bible study on the epistle of James at his childhood church, Trinity Baptist. Ann turned the note pages for him. He occasionally preached at a Baptist church in the small town of Drain, Oregon.

The Brownings continued to attend Valley Hills as regular members. An interim minister served for about a year until Dan Brandel became the full-time pastor. Larry filled in occasionally.

Ann, a short and petite woman, had been Larry's full-time caregiver since he lost function of both legs in 2003. She bathed him in the mornings and put him to bed at night. Larry, 5' 11", had developed a paunch from inactivity. So, this tiny woman had to regularly move a fairly large man. When he lost most of the use of his arms, Ann's load became overwhelming.

In 2006, her parents, Bob and Margaret Kintigh, offered to pay for a caregiver to work three mornings a week. The Brownings accepted the gift and hired a man named Gary, who cared for Larry for about a year.

When Gary was first hired, Larry could still lift his right arm enough to feed himself. By the end of the 2006, others had to feed him. He could move his right hand enough to operate the toggle of the electric wheelchair. Another caregiver, Evan, replaced Gary in 2007.

Larry's stepfather, Lynn Morse, passed away from a stroke in February, 2007. At the time of his death, he had been battling pancreatic cancer. At the funeral, Larry gave a heartfelt presentation covering Lynn's life. Agatha, now widowed twice, faced a triple burden of grief—for Jay, Lynn, and her steadily declining son.

The MS progressed slowly throughout 2007 and 2008. However, a problem indirectly related to the disease hit Larry hard during this period. Harsh memories of the Vietnam War plagued him like never before.

His symptoms of post-traumatic stress disorder (PTSD) first began to surface in 2003. The Second Gulf War began then, and Larry felt disturbed by the similarities and differences between the wars in Iraq and Vietnam. Both wars were unpopular with the general public, but GI's returning from Iraq were treated much better than Vietnam veterans. Larry was glad about the favorable welcome given the Iraq vets. However, psychological wounds resurfaced concerning the bad treatment Vietnam vets had received.

Also in 2003, Larry lost any remaining use of his legs, and he spent all waking hours in the wheelchair. Less physical distractions resulted in more time to think about the war.

His retirement in 2005 resulted in less time to prepare sermons and more time to think. In 2006, he lost most of the use of his arms and hands, reducing physical activity even more.

By 2007, Larry found himself with huge chunks of time to sit and think. Day in and day out, he sat. Weeks of sitting. Months of sitting. The painful memories of Vietnam weighed on him with full force.

In his mind, Larry continually replayed the day of the ambush that left four men dead. He vividly pictured Clarence lying on the ground with the back of his head blown off. The horror of the event hit Larry with immediacy, as if it just happened.

Larry had always wanted to contact Clarence's family to explain what happened the day of the ambush. During the 1970's he tried to forget about the war by smoking a lot of dope, so he had postponed the painful phone call to the family. And throughout his active years of ministry he continued to deny the wounds that existed deep in his psyche over the Vietnam War.

Says Ann, "I think Larry's mode of operation, with all the hard things he's been through in his life, is to stuff things. I think he had totally stuffed Vietnam. I think he stuffed his dad's death. I think he stuffed Karen's [death]."

Larry attempted to contact Clarence's family, probably in 2007. He first spoke to Clarence's aunt, who gave him the phone number of the parents.

"So I called them," he says, "and told them that I had a picture of Clarence because he came into the company the same day I did. I thought they might want that. And so they said they'd like me to send it, but they didn't want to hear anything about how he'd gotten killed or anything. I wrote them a letter, put the picture in it, gave my number and said, 'If you ever want to talk, give me a call.' I never heard anything from them. I guess, from what the aunt said, they were still very bitter about the war. Again, Clarence was expecting a child who he never saw."

At the time of this writing (February 2011), Larry still analyzes and reanalyzes the details of the ambush. He thinks he could have done something to prevent it. After all, just minutes before, he and Ace had shot at a straggler, probably a member of the VC ambush team. Larry now asks himself why he hadn't better assessed the situation and warned his company—or personally done something to prevent the attack.

There are some logical problems with Larry's efforts to

blame himself. First, his company, on the trail just ahead, would have heard the loud shots he and Ace fired at the straggler. The gunfire would have provided plenty of warning that the enemy was near. Second, both Ace and the platoon sergeant were also aware of the straggler. They were superior to Larry in both rank and experience. If anything could have been done to prevent the ambush, they were in a much better position than Larry to do something about it.

Survivor's guilt often accompanies post-traumatic stress disorder, which may explain Larry's efforts at self-blame.

Another problem arose in 2007. While reading the newspaper, Ann discovered some shocking information. Someone had filed a $375,000 lawsuit against the Brownings and an additional $300,000 suit against Valley Hills Community Church. The person claimed to have suffered an injury from Larry's van accident in 2004.

Says Ann, "I thought we were going to lose everything. We settled out of court. They put a lien against the house, which went away when he [Larry] died. Because he was the driver, they didn't name me in the suit."

A generous neighbor paid the Brownings' attorney's fees. The settlement was limited to the lien, so Ann and Larry were spared any financial burden. Says Ann, "I mean, the things that God provided. We were living on $1229 a month then. We couldn't pay an attorney."

In 2008, a VA psychiatrist diagnosed Larry with PTSD. The Brownings received appropriate benefits, even a refund for past medical co-payments. The extra income enabled them to afford additional home care for Larry. This helped lighten the physical burden on Ann, though her heart continued to break over Larry's deterioration.

Ann describes every stage of Larry's decline as the

worst. "Each stage is really awful. I remember at the very beginning they gave us a metal frame to [help] put on his stockings. And we're like, 'This is so awful not to be able to put on your socks.' And that's like the worst thing ever. But then as you go along, the stage before sounds pretty good. Not being able to put on your socks sounds really good."

The Brownings decided that they would do their best to keep Larry at home as long as possible. This hinged on whether Ann could bear up under the physical and emotional burden. If the pressure broke her, Larry would have to live at a care facility.

Says Ann, "For the last two years [2010-11], everyday I didn't think I could make it the next day. I just prayed all the time. I remember praying that he would live till Paige graduated from high school, and that I could keep him home till then. It would have been awful for him to be somewhere else."

How did she find strength to endure?

"It was God," she says. "It was God…because I'm not a caregiver person. God's word becomes so alive and I'm so struck by that… He is so real and so alive in His promises."

What did she struggle with most during Larry's illness? "Can I say 'everything'? I think it's that loneliness and the loss of the dream. Not being able to have the physical closeness. You just don't understand, I think, until you're there. You can't separate the caregiving thing, and I'm old-fashioned in that I'm one that wants my husband to take care of me and that sort of thing. So that's just all a changed course."

Ann mentions how wheelchair inaccessibility contributed to the loneliness. "You can't go to most people's houses. We couldn't even go to sit at [some] family members' houses."

Even in church, isolation affected both Ann and Larry. When he lost the use of his hands, he couldn't move around and mix with people, or search for particular individuals. People needed to approach him. Ann couldn't drift away from Larry for long. If he wanted to talk to a particular person, Ann's job was to track them down.

In January 2008, the Brownings began attending McKenzie Bible Fellowship (MBF), a Conservative Baptist church, conveniently located just five minutes from their rural home. Larry had gotten to know some of the members through an early-morning men's Bible study he'd attended a few years before.

Fifteen-year-old Paige was less than enthusiastic about the change. "I was against it more than you can be against anything else. I fought my parents tooth and nail. I did not want to leave [Valley Hills Community Church], because it was all I had ever known. That church was my heart and soul. I loved Valley Hills and I still love the people there."

Paige asked her parents if she could attend Valley Hills on her own. They said no and pointed to scripture that stated, "Honor your father and mother." Paige submitted, though she remained angry at them for a while.

At this time, Ryan, a student at Oregon State University, felt the horrible reality of his father's condition. As Larry entered the latter stages of the disease, Ryan often questioned God. "I didn't understand why he had MS. It seemed so unfair for him to suffer."

Ryan sometimes experienced hurt when around friends. "It was hard for me to hear my friends talk about all the things they did with their parents. I also felt pretty alone a lot of the time because none of my friends had any idea of what I was going through."

Though his heart ached during high school and college, Ryan explains how his faith in God grew stronger: "By watching how his [Larry's] faith got stronger and stronger as his condition got worse and worse, he showed me what it means to continue to praise God in any situation. He also showed me what it meant to trust God with every aspect of my life. He had a very strong impact on my faith. When I went away to college, my faith stayed strong mostly because of him."

When the Brownings had attended McKenzie Bible Fellowship a short time, Pastor Dick Roberts invited Larry to preach. He accepted and gave his testimony. Soon, he and Ann began attending a Wednesday evening Bible study.

Larry often accompanied a group of men from MBF, who ministered once a month at the Eugene Mission. He sometimes gave the main message during the chapel service.

In 2009, Larry began losing sight in his left eye; and the fingers of his right hand began to fail, making it difficult to operate the electric wheelchair. His right eye still functioned normally.

That summer, I became his caregiver five mornings per week, replacing Evan. In September, Larry traveled to Seattle with some friends to watch a Mariners/Yankees baseball game. It was the last live sporting event he would be able to see.

By the end of 2009, his right eye also began to fail; and he could no longer move his right hand the two inches needed to operate the toggle on his wheelchair. He and Ann decided to replace the heavy electric wheelchair with a lightweight, easy-to-push model.

James 5:14-15 (ESV) states, "Is anyone among you sick? Let him call for the elders of the church, and let them pray over him, anointing him with oil in the name of the Lord. And the prayer of faith will save the one who is sick, and the Lord will raise him up."

Larry did not interpret the James passage as an absolute promise for healing. He saw it as a biblical guideline on how to pray for those who are sick. In early December of 2009, he asked the elders of McKenzie Bible Fellowship to pray for him and anoint his head with oil. He believed that a healing would be a great way to give God glory. It would be a testimony to the community. Most of the elders met at the Browning home and prayed for Larry, anointing his head with oil.

Healing did not occur. Larry began 2010 completely quadriplegic and nearly blind.

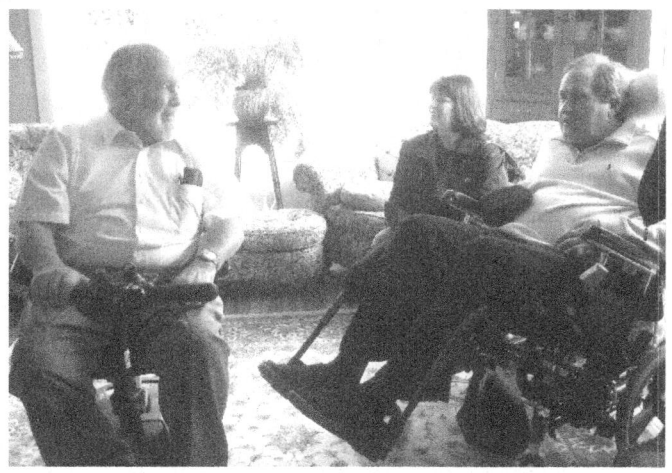

With father-in-law Bob Kintigh. March 2010.

As a last-ditch effort to reverse the MS-caused blindness, his doctor prescribed high doses of prednisone for one week in January 2010. With his left-eye vision gone and his right vision reduced to blurs, Larry figured it couldn't hurt. But it did. Throughout the week, he experienced the following side effects: extreme anxiety, depression, anger, profuse sweating and insomnia.

"When you can't sleep and can't move your arms and legs, it feels like you're buried alive in a coffin," he said. Larry made the best of the sleeplessness and spent most of those hours praying for everyone and everything he could think of. He exhibited some rare grouchiness that week. The prednisone proved ineffective and he vowed never to take it again.

With his vision reduced to blurs of light and shadow, Larry began hallucinating. "When I'm at home," he said, "[the hallucinations] are generally just in the morning when I first wake up. I see this paisley pattern all over my room. It's even on the caregiver when he comes in the morning. But when I was in respite care at South Hills [August 2010], it was an all-day experience. One morning I woke up—I'd been having a dream—and the people that were in my dream were standing at the foot of my bed. When the caregiver came in, she looked like one of the people in my dream. That probably lasted thirty seconds to a minute and then they disappeared."

Larry easily distinguished the hallucinations from reality and none were scary. "I've kind of gotten used to them," he said, describing the figments as, at worst, a nuisance. He only saw them when his eyes were open. Closing his eyes gave relief, so they didn't interfere with his sleep.

His doctor speculated that MS lesions on the vision centers of his brain may have caused the hallucinations. Also, hallucinations can be a side effect of the drug Nortriptyline, which Larry took to prevent fiery leg pain.

Larry began receiving hospice care in September 2010. His doctor estimated he had about a year to live. His breathing was getting weaker and his ability to swallow would likely be the next thing to fail.

Larry's advance directive prohibited the use of unnatural means to keep him alive. "I don't want any feeding tubes or any life support of any kind," he said on September 29, 2010. "If my swallowing did get too bad where I couldn't eat, I'm sure it would be a matter of time to where my kidneys would quit functioning and I would probably die. But I'm ready to die because I know where I'm going."

At this time Larry stopped taking Azathioprine, a drug known to slow the progression of MS. A VA nurse told him that without it, the MS would likely progress faster. Larry doubted that Azathioprine or any of the other drugs had ever slowed the disease.

His ability to swallow failed to worsen after five months, so at the end of February 2011, the doctor took him off hospice.

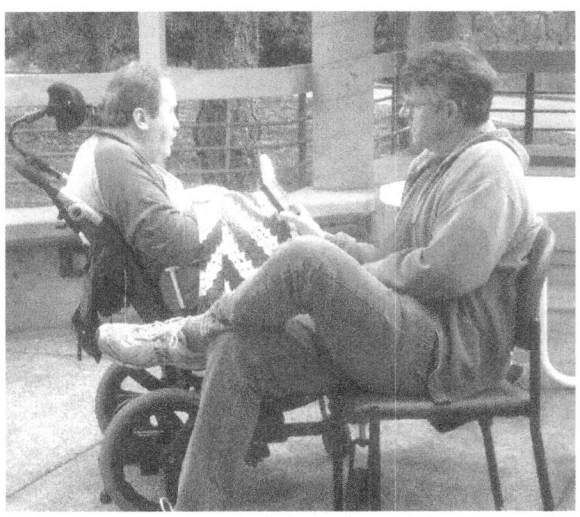

At Roseburg VA, being interviewed by Tom. April 2011

One morning in March, Larry could barely talk, and he answered questions with mumbles. His blood pressure was normal and his temperature read 96.9. His urine was somewhat cloudy. Ann called the VA. The doctor speculated that Larry may have had a stroke and should visit the ER.

"No," said Larry, without mumbling. "I'll take my chances."

"That's what I thought you'd say," said Ann. "How do you feel?"

"I feel fine," said Larry. "I'm not going to pay $800 to find out nothing's wrong."

His speech and attentiveness returned to normal by the end of the day. A nurse speculated that the cloudy urine may have indicated a urinary tract infection, which can sometimes cause disorientation.

In May 2011, Paige arrived home from California Baptist University where she studied nursing. She would spend the summer with her parents.

By mid-May, Larry had stopped taking several meds. He only took those which alleviated pain and other negative symptoms of MS. He now swallowed only six pills, three times a day, instead of twelve.

His hallucinations stopped at this time, along with his ability to see any light. Total blindness had set in.

A rainy spring ended and summer began. Larry's breathing had declined to where he often couldn't speak. He'd be talkative and alert one day, sleepy and silent the next. He slept more during the day, sometimes dozing off in the middle of breakfast. Pizza, one of his favorite foods, now tasted like cardboard. His appetite decreased, but his thirst increased. He guzzled water like never before. Incontinence set in.

Larry went back on hospice in July 2011. The doctor estimated his life expectancy at less than a year. The hospice nurse told Ann that when people are unable to communicate, they tend to pass away fairly soon. But the nurse couldn't tell Ann *how* soon.

Agatha struggled greatly as these new symptoms emerged. She wept often during this time. She phoned one day and asked me how her son was. He'd been silent that morning and was napping. She cried and said how hard it was watching him slowly go.

Dick Roberts, the pastor of McKenzie Bible Fellowship, had a meeting with Larry in mid-July. They discussed the funeral. Larry asked Dick to give a clear presentation of the gospel during the service.

Larry's sister, Brenda, traveled from North Carolina to spend time with her brother. She stayed for two weeks at Agatha's home in Springfield, some twenty miles away.

Larry had a talkative day on August 2. When I asked him what he'd been thinking about during the last few weeks, he said, "Well, I've had mixed feelings about it." On the plus side, he felt pleased that the end was near. The downside was that his symptoms and quality of life had now reached a low point. He mentioned, again, his immense disappointment at losing his sight, noting how it prevented good communication with his family. He talked about Vietnam and rehashed his feeling that he should have done something to prevent the ambush. Again, I told him he shouldn't blame himself, because if the ambush could have been prevented, Ace and the sergeant were in a better position to do so.

Larry's frequent silences didn't mean he lacked awareness. He always said yes when asked if he understood the conversations around him.

Caregiving lacked predictability at this time. Larry's recent needs required a new set of tasks. I often had to figure things out on the fly. At times Larry would break his silence to offer good suggestions.

This silent phase of Larry's life made the heartache worse for his loved ones. He had always been the one to start and carry conversations. It was now up to the rest of us to offer him good company and speak words that would edify and comfort him as he neared the end.

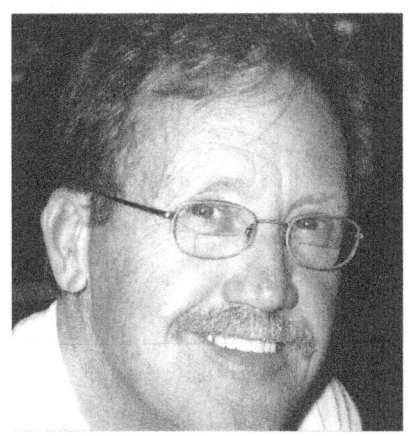

Modern-day Job?

ഇൗരു

14
HAVE YOU CONSIDERED
MY SERVANT LARRY?

Pastor Dick Roberts holds open the door to Aunt Ding's Restaurant, a popular family eatery in the McKenzie River valley. I wheel Larry inside, past the *Please Seat Yourself* sign. The cozy restaurant is decorated like a country home, with white lace valances over the windows and antique copper kitchenware adorning high shelves. Local art is displayed on the walls. But most importantly, the pleasant smell of bacon and eggs wafts through the air.

It's just before ten o'clock and the early morning breakfast rush has passed. The three of us sit at a table in the middle of the dining area and I adjust the wheelchair so Larry's thighs are low enough to slide under the square tabletop. Local folks, truckers, and retirees populate the room, and they're good about not gawking at the guy in the wheelchair.

I'm no multitasker, but on this June morning, 2010, I'll feed Larry breakfast, feed myself and try to lead a three-way discussion on the biblical book of Job.

Dick Roberts, pastor of McKenzie Bible Fellowship, earned a Ph.D. in Biblical Studies from Louisiana Baptist University in Shreveport and a Master of Theology from Western Seminary in Portland. He majored in Old Testament and taught Biblical Hebrew for three years as a teaching fellow at Western Seminary.

Larry brings to the table twenty years of pastoral experience and exceptional wisdom learned from a lifetime of loss and suffering. He's a modern-day Job.

For those readers unfamiliar with the story of Job, it's about a wealthy, blameless and godly man who underwent great loss and suffering at the hands of Satan. God permitted Satan to strip away Job's land, wealth and possessions; kill his children and servants; and physically torment him with sickness, painful boils and other afflictions. God gave Satan one restriction, "…only spare his life." (Job 2:6 ESV)

We settle into our seats and small talk ensues. Larry reminisces about a hard-drinking uncle and a quirky grandmother. The story is interrupted by the hostess, Lori, who arrives with menus and a pot of hot coffee.

I slide three of Larry's fingers through his coffee mug handle and position his arm near his chest so the straw is near his lips.

"Fill'r up," says Larry.

"All the way, darlin'," says Lori. She fills Larry's mug, then mine. Dick passes.

Lori moves to the next table and Larry resumes. "Yeah,

my grandmother was 104 when she died. She dipped snuff."

"Maybe we should all do that," I say.

"If you get enough bad stuff in your body, the germs can't survive," says Dick.

Larry smiles, finishes his story and asks me what's on the menu. I read from the list of classic, all-American diner fare mixed with a few of Aunt Ding's originals. We ponder today's special, the Italian omelet.

A waitress arrives. "Are you getting close, guys?"

"I'm ready," says Dick. He orders a Farmer's Tater scramble with white toast.

The waitress delivers an enticing pitch for the Italian omelet, but Larry opts for a ham and cheese omelet with two pancakes. I order a Denver omelet.

"What's your name?" Larry asks her.

"I'm Bobbie Jo," she says and scoots toward the kitchen until she's out of earshot from us.

"That's a country name," says Larry. "Sounds like she's out of Texas."

I put on my best announcer's voice. "Our waitress is Bobbie Jo."

"Bobbie Jo," chuckles Dick, "serving an Italian omelet."

We spend a few more seconds musing over the cosmic implications of Bobbie Jo's name, then I suggest we get down to business.

Larry starts us off. "You know, as we talk about Job, at the very beginning, the doctrine of God's sovereignty is established, because Satan had to ask for permission."

"Right," says Dick, "And there were limits on what he was allowed to do." Dick describes the first two chapters as providing crucial background for the rest of the book. These opening sections contain the dialogue between God and Satan, and the two-phased afflictions that hit Job in a short space of time.

Over the last few days, Larry had been listening to the book of Job on CD. He confesses to finding the lengthy middle section—containing the endless speeches of Job's three friends—to be rather sleep-inducing. "They were bloviating," says Larry. "They just like to hear themselves talk."

Dick offers his take on the long, poetic monologues that fill the middle of the book. "You've got three friends [Eliphaz, Bildad, Zophar] and Job speaking. They go through these cycles where they speak and then he defends himself. I really think what they're saying is, 'Job, the reason you're suffering is that there's some sin in your life.' Job's response is, 'If that's the case, show me what it is.' He even asks God to show him what it is and God won't accommodate him—God won't answer him. So, I see Job and the three friends working off the same basis: assuming that suffering comes as a result of sin in one's life."

Larry agrees. "Even in the New Testament, that was an assumption, that if you were ill or something, it was due to sin."

He mentions the incident where Jesus heals the man born blind. "The disciples asked, 'Rabbi, who sinned, this man or his parents, that he was born blind?' Jesus answered, 'It was not that this man sinned, or his parents, but that the works of God might be displayed in him.'" (John 9:2-3 ESV)

I add, "Now, Job, because he's on that same premise, is questioning God's integrity."

"Yes," says Dick, "and he also assumes God is angry with him. In fact, in one verse [Job says], 'He set me up as his target.'" (Job 16:12 ESV)

As our discussion warms up, Bobbie Jo arrives with the meals and Lori follows with coffee. The restaurant crowd is a bit sparse, with only a few folks eating late breakfasts. I pray over the meal and the discussion continues.

Dick mentions God's silence from chapter three through thirty-seven. "Job really wants God to give an account for why he's suffering, and God's not cooperating. And that's part of the frustration."

"And God never does give him the explanation," I say, trying to feed Larry a bite of omelet. The chunks of ham keep falling off the fork. "It seems to me, on the surface, it's simply a wager between God and Satan. God kind of entices Satan and says, 'Consider my servant Job, a righteous man.' Then Satan says, 'You take away blessing and cause suffering—and Job will curse you to your face.'"

"A divine wager," says Dick. "I think what's behind it, though, is when God makes a wager, you know who's going to win. Behind it all is that no matter what Satan brings into Job's life, God will give him whatever he needs to overcome it. Job never does curse God to his face, and I don't think it was because Job's strength was so great."

Larry interrupts to give me instructions. "Just give me my omelet first."

"Then the pancakes second?" I ask.

He nods. Maybe he considers the pancakes dessert.

As I fumble with Larry's meal, Dick offers some background information, explaining that the book of Job was likely written during the time of Abraham. "There are no references to Israel or Jacob. There are other ancient near-Eastern literatures that have similar stories about a suffering, righteous person. So, Job may have been an actual historical figure who was well known by other people in that time."

Bobbi Joe approaches our table. "Is everybody doing okay over here?"

"Yes, thank you," says Larry.

We continue with the question of why God willed for Job to suffer. We establish that it was not due to his sin. After all, God said in the first chapter, "There is no one on earth like him; he is blameless and upright, a man who fears God and shuns evil." (Job 1:8 NIV)

Dick offers another possibility for God's motives. "You might say it was God flexing his arm."

"Doing what?" asks Larry.

"Flexing his arm—especially against Satan, who challenged Him in the first place."

Dick's comment is similar to what I'd read in the *Christian Workers' Commentary on the Whole Bible* by James M. Gray, D.D. (Spire Books, 1977). I share my findings. "The premise is that the test was not actually for Job. The test was for God—whether God was going to uphold Job and help him not give in and maintain his integrity throughout. It was a test of God's power to enable Job to do that."

"I think that's a good point," says Dick, "because in the very beginning, Satan's challenge really isn't against Job, it's against God."

"So in a way it should increase our faith that God has the power to get us through anything," I say, then shovel a big bite of the Denver omelet in my mouth.

"Like in your case, Larry," says Dick. "Part of Job's frustration is God won't tell him why he's suffering. So, as your disease deteriorated, you must have had those same questions; I don't know if you did or not."

"Yeah," says Larry. "My question is more, 'God, why haven't you healed me?' I pray consistently; I've just asked God to give me my eyesight back. My right eye is blind, my left eye is real hazy. I've told God, 'God, I would certainly like you to heal me, so I could do things with my kids, with my wife.' I've said,

'If you're not going to heal me physically, then why don't you just let me go home?' There are times, after sitting in this chair day in and day out, being unable to see…I listen to tapes, but a lot of times I fall asleep, I'll sleep for three or four hours in the afternoon. So it seems pointless that I'm really not doing a lot. Not only is this a hardship for me, it's a hardship for my wife, because she feels like I do, she's kind of trapped. She gets lonely."

Bobbie Jo comes by and fills my coffee cup. She asks Larry, "Do you need any more in your cup?"

"Please," says Larry. She fills it and he thanks her.

"You're welcome," she says.

Dick points out a similarity between Ann Browning and Job's wife, that they endure(d) hardships because of their husbands' sufferings. "She [Job's wife] lost her children, she lost her home. Job's suffering extended to her as well."

I share what I learned from an audio teaching by Chuck Smith in the Blue Letter Bible website. "When she [Job's wife] said, 'Curse God and die,' she was actually feeling sorry for Job. It sounds as if she's being obnoxious when you first read it, but she was actually looking out for his welfare."

"In the midst of my affliction," says Larry, "I've never come to a point where I felt like cursing God. One of the things I acknowledge on a daily basis is that He's the potter and I'm the clay—and He can do with me what He wills. He didn't necessarily cause the disease. It's the result of a fallen world. As Isaiah said, 'It rains on the just as well as the unjust.' So I just pray, 'Lord, heal me, if it be Thy will. If not, shorten Your timetable and get me out of here.'"

Dick laughs, and I smile at Larry's brash petition.

I ask, "Have you been *tempted* to curse God? Have you felt like it?"

"No," answers Larry. "I've never questioned God, except when my first wife died. I asked God, "Why?" because there seemed to be no logical answer. She was 38 years old. She was enjoying life...."

Larry perceives that Dick is attempting to pay for our meals. "Hey, Dick, I'm going to pay for all that."

"Pay for what, the meal?" says Dick, caught in the act.

"The food," says Larry.

"You are?" says Dick.

I assert my generosity. "Naw, I am."

Dick laughs. "You are?"

"Yeah," I say. "I'm the one who pushed for this meeting."

They concede.

Larry continues. "I'm not really blaming God. I've never really asked God why He's allowed this to happen. I don't think God *caused* it to happen, I think He *allowed* it to happen because of His sovereignty."

"God can do what God wants to do," says Dick.

"But there's a reason why He hasn't healed me. Because of my illness and my help from the VA, I'm able to give more money to missions and to the church than I've ever given before. God has really blessed us financially in the midst of all this."

Larry has said this before when asked how his illness has worked for the good. His answer of financial blessing always falls flat to me. I don't tell him this, but it seems to me that God would need to bless him with, say, a billion dollars to compensate for all the misery he's gone through. Sure, the Brownings are able to save a little now, but it's not all that much.

Dick asks, "Have you gone through a period in your life where you wondered, 'Is it something I've done that the Lord has caused this?'"

"I've wondered if my past had anything to do with it," says Larry, "because when I was twenty-one, I openly told God that I knew the right path, but I was going to follow the path of sin, because it looked good. So I openly rebelled against God for seven to ten years, at least."

Dick probes. "How would you explain other people having similar rebellious periods in their life, but not having been afflicted like you have?"

Larry responds. "Paul said in Romans, 'There is no condemnation for those who are in Christ Jesus.' So I don't think God would punish me for the sins of the past."

"Exactly," says Dick. "Yeah, yeah."

I venture a theory. "Could it be that just the opposite is true? That God caused/allowed Job's suffering *because* he was a good man? He was the prime example of how good a human being could be in that day and age. If Job had more flaws, maybe God wouldn't have used him."

Bobbie Joe drifts our way. "Can I get those out of the way for ya?"

"Sure, thanks," I say. She busses some of our plates.

Lori comes by with more coffee. "How about Larry; does Larry want more coffee?"

"Yeah," he says, "might as well."

Larry can't reach his coffee mug straw, so I readjust it closer to his mouth.

"Boy," says Dick, "you guys serve a lot of coffee."

"Yeah, we do," says Lori, moving to the next table.

Dick continues, "Job is presented as the godliest man on earth. The point that God proved is that no matter what Satan brings against God's servants, they have the strength within to overcome it. We know that comes from the Lord. But the whole thing with Job, which is similar to what you experience, is that

God didn't give him any answers. You can guess, you can think, and you can see some good that comes out of it. But the reality of it is, in a lot of aspects of our life, he simply doesn't tell us why he does what he does. At that point we're left to either trust him or walk away from him. But he's not accountable. We don't like that, we want people to give an account for what they do."

"Walking away from God," says Larry, "that alternative is not very good. I think of the verse that says it's better to go lame and blind into the kingdom of God, than to dwell in the tents of the wicked [Matthew 18:8-9]. One thing is, I think a lot more about heaven now than I did when I was in good health."

Dick chuckles. "I'm sure you do."

"And I'm a lot more eager to get there. When I get to heaven, it would be like Helen Keller said—that the first person she hoped to see would be the Lord Jesus."

"What keeps you going from day to day?" asks Dick.

"The Lord has given me the strength," says Larry. "If it weren't for the Lord, I would have opted for assisted suicide a long time ago. But because I know the Lord is in control and that he's determined all my days, I'm not going to do anything like that, because that's the Lord's place, not mine." He turns to me. "Can I have another bite?"

"Sorry, Larry." It's been a few minutes since I've fed him. I quickly cut a piece of pancake, dip it in maple syrup, and fork it into his mouth.

Dick brings up chapters 38-41, where the Lord speaks out of the whirlwind and rebukes Job for his contention of being treated unjustly. God fires question after question at Job, who answers, "Behold, I am of small account; what shall I answer you?" (Job 40:4 ESV) God then barrages Job with more questions until Job repents, saying, "I know that you can do all things, and that no purpose of yours can be thwarted." (Job 42:2 ESV)

"There comes a point," says Dick, "where you say, 'The Lord's chosen not to heal me. The Lord's chosen not to answer me. Lord, do whatever You need to do, even though I don't know what the purpose is.' But God doesn't do anything without purpose."

"When I get to heaven," says Larry, "it won't matter what the purpose was. You know, I just think about my first glimpse of God, Who spoke the universe into being. I can't even imagine that you could do anything but fall on your face before Him."

Lori stops by our table. "Any more coffee?"

"No thank you," says Larry.

I nod yes.

"You're gonna float," says Lori, filling my mug.

"Thanks, that's good," I say.

"I'm ready for the rest of that, Tom," says Larry, eyeing his pancake.

"Oh, yeah," I say.

In an attempt at multitasking, I feed Larry more pancake and ask Dick a question at the same time. "J. Vernon McGee made a point that Job was self-righteous. Do you think Job was self-righteous in a prideful sense?"

Dick flips through his notes and reads from Job 32-35, where a fifth character, young Elihu, arrives and says to Job, "I have heard the sound of your words: 'I [Job] am pure, without transgression; I'm innocent and there is no guilt in me. Behold, He [God] invents pretexts against me. He counts me as His enemy.'" (Job 33:9-10 NASB) And in Job 35:2, Elihu says, "Do you say, 'My righteousness is more than God's?'"

Says Dick, "His [Elihu's] indictment is that Job is justifying himself at the expense of God's righteousness. The three friends accused Job of wrong-doing, but couldn't provide any evidence. He [Elihu] says to them 'Indeed, there was no one who refuted Job, not one of you who answered his words.' (Job 32:12 NASB)

"His [Elihu's] response to Job is, 'Shall God recompense you on your terms?' (Job 34:33 NASB) [Elihu critiques] this idea that God needs to answer our questions, that we set the terms for what God can do and what God can't do."

Says Larry, "What I've come to is God can do whatever He wants to, and I need to be submissive to that."

"So in a way, Elihu is correct?" I ask.

"He is," says Dick. "Out of the five speakers in the book of Job, the Lord rebukes four of them. Elihu is simply not mentioned. His judgment is that God is high and exalted and we can't figure Him out. The last thing he says, 'The Almighty—we cannot find Him; He is exalted in power; and He will not do violence to justice and abundant righteousness. Therefore men fear Him. He does not regard any who are wise of heart.' (Job 37:23-24 NASB) There are secret things that the Lord holds to Himself, then there are things that are revealed. Sometimes God chooses not to reveal His secrets. That's His prerogative to do."

Dick continues. "Another subtle theme of the book of Job, is that we can't comprehend God. He's beyond. He's high and mighty. He does things we don't understand. It's almost like there's mystery about God that we have to submit to, because He's not accountable to us. We don't have the right to demand answers. If He chooses to give us answers, it's because of His choice at that point."

"He wouldn't be God," says Larry, "if He were accountable to us. My question is not why, but how long? How long am I going to have to endure this, God? Having pastored almost twenty years, I've certainly come to the place where I believe in the total sovereignty of God."

Larry tells the story of Whitworth University professor Jerry Sittser, whose wife, mother and four-year-old daughter died in a car accident caused by a drunk driver. In his book, *A Grace Disguised* (Zondervan 2004), Sittser describes how he initially despaired because of the sense of randomness and unfairness of the tragedy. He and his family did nothing to deserve such loss.

But later, Sittser concluded that he would much rather take his chances in an unfair world, because if we received everything in life based on fairness, we could never hope to obtain God's incredible blessings given by grace (unmerited favor).

Says Larry, "As the Potter, God can do whatever He wants. He pours out his mercy and grace, but also He sometimes meets us with justice. The bottom line is that I don't deserve anything from God. And I'm just thankful that God chose me before the foundation of the earth, to be found in Him. I know that when my life does come to an end, that I'm going to be with Him for all eternity."

While God blesses us based on His mercy and grace, there are other times when He rewards us for obedience. Says Dick, "I do think there's a relationship between the suffering we endure here on earth for the sake of the Lord and the glory that we will enjoy eternally in the presence of the Lord. Peter talks about it, that those who suffer are going to be rewarded to a [greater] degree [than] those that have chosen not to suffer for the sake of Christ."

"I sometimes question whether or not my suffering is for the Lord," responds Larry.

Many Christians suffer specifically for the cause of Christ; they're persecuted for proclaiming their faith or even killed as martyrs. Larry wasn't "persecuted" with multiple sclerosis. MS doesn't discriminate between Christians and non-

Christians, good people or bad people. It just happens. So it's a fair question whether or not he's suffering for the Lord.

Dick responds. "Well, I think [suffering can be for the Lord] even if it's just submitting to the suffering, as opposed to shaking your fist at God and turning against Him or complaining against Him."

Bobbie Jo comes by with coffee. I finally tell her no.

"Do you identify with the book of Job?" asks Dick.

"To some degree," says Larry. "Sometimes I can identify with him in the suffering, but I think I've suffered a lot longer than Job did. And I don't think God's going to heal me, although I don't know that. I've never had friends like Job's come over and tell me I'm a sinner."

Larry speculates that he, like Job, may be part of a wager between God and Satan:

"I wonder if God said, 'Have you considered my servant, Larry?' I don't know if that happened; I like to think that it did. You know, Satan is zero for two."

Larry wants more coffee, so I flag down Bobbie Jo.

She arrives. "Both you guys want more coffee?"

"Just Larry," I say. Then I change my mind. "Half a mug for me, I guess."

Job endured two attacks by Satan. First, Satan took all his possessions and the lives of his children. "The second one," says Dick, "he [Satan] comes back and says [to God], 'Skin for skin, everything a man possesses he'll give for his health.' (Job 2:4) Then he takes his health away. We do regard our health as of greater value than material things."

"Oh yeah," says Larry. "You know how people say, 'Your health is everything.' I'd rather have my health than all the money in the world."

"Would you trade your health for your family?" asks

Dick.

"No," answers Larry.

"So, for Christians in particular," says Dick. "we would hold our families as of greater value to us than our health. Our relationship with Christ—we would give up our health for that. So, our life isn't at the top of the list."

I ask, "What is meant in Job 2:3, when God says to Satan, 'He still holds fast his integrity, although you incited me against him to destroy him without reason.'? Did God Himself directly afflict Job? We know that Satan did a certain amount, but it sounds here that God claims to have done it."

"Ultimately," says Dick, "God called the shots, so to speak."

"Yeah," agrees Larry.

Dick elaborates. "Satan became an instrument in God's hand to bring this affliction into Job's life. Satan tries to use it to get Job to sin. God's going to use it to show His power, His sovereignty, His authority. But Satan didn't work independent of God in this. This isn't Satan's sovereignty on display here. This is God's sovereignty."

"So in a sense," I say, "it was God's will for this to happen."

"Yeah," says Dick. "Since Satan issued the challenge, the Lord says, 'Okay, I'll take the hedge away from him, and you do whatever you want to him.' So, Satan couldn't come back to say, 'Well, You were too easy on him.' He let Satan do as much as Satan could do."

The restaurant is now busy with the lunchtime crowd. People around us seem relaxed in conversation, upbeat. Good food does that. A child prattles loudly; dishes clatter; a phone rings. Bobbie Joe's laughter carries through the air. The diners are a mix of families, truckers, travelers and retirees—lots of blue jeans, plaid shirts and baseball caps.

"Ultimately," says Dick, "it's that question of any evil. Who's responsible for it? Could God eliminate evil if He so chooses? And He could, if He's all powerful and all sovereign."

"And He will," says Larry.

Dick agrees. "But it's allowed to continue because there are certain aspects of God's character that are seen against the background of evil. Were the evil not here, you wouldn't know that there is mercy from God. You wouldn't know there is judgment from God. Were it not for the presence of evil, there are certain aspects of God's character that would be unseen."

The book of Job contains a number of quotations by Satan and seemingly endless quotations by Job's three friends. These characters often speak falsehoods, sometimes lies. It's safe to say they are not reliable sources of truth. The question of biblical inerrancy arises. Does inerrancy mean that everything written in the Bible is true?

Dick offers some clarity. "All that inerrancy attempts to guarantee is the accuracy of what was recorded. There are lies recorded in the Bible; they are an accurate record of what was said. You just have to make sure you see them in context as falsehoods."

"Also," I say, "inerrancy means that not only is it accurately recorded, but it's inspired."

"God-breathed," says Larry.

"Yeah," says Dick. "Yes."

"It is inspired and accurately recorded—but it might be a lie," I say, chuckling at the seeming incongruity. The thought of a holy God, who calls Himself "the Truth," purposely including inspired lies in His Word—it just seems wrong. But it's true. The first lie occurred in Genesis 3, when the serpent tempted Eve to eat fruit from the tree of the knowledge of good and evil. He lied to Eve, saying, "You surely shall not die!" (Genesis 3:4 NASB). Previously, God had made it clear that she and Adam would die if they ate from the tree.

Bobbie Joe walks by. "Any more coffee, guys?"

"No, we're fine," says Larry.

Dick continues. "That's why you can't just cherry-pick verses out of the Bible because they seem to fit your argument—because you could be choosing a verse that's not true. It's truly recorded, but the statement might be false. But the things that did find their way in the Bible are there because God made a conscious choice to include them in the Scripture."

Our breakfasts are history. Two-and-a-half hours have passed since we arrived.

"Does this wear you out?" Dick asks Larry. "Are you getting tired, talking a lot?"

"No," says Larry, "I'll probably go to sleep when I get home. I enjoy it, to be honest with you."

I'm amazed at Larry's stamina. He's usually zonked out after just a half hour of conversation.

"But if you had your druthers," asks Dick. "would you rather be with the Lord than sitting here?"

"I'd rather be healed physically. Paige has already lost her mother. We're so close and I think it would be harder on her than anybody. Being here, even in this condition, is better for her than for me to be in heaven."

"So there is some purpose for you being here," says Dick.

"Paige and I talked about it just the other day. I didn't bring it up, and she told me, 'Dad, if the Lord took you home, I would be devastated. But I know that the Lord would see me through it.'"

And the Lord *will* see Paige through it, just like he saw

Job through his trials.

There are many lessons to be learned from the sufferings of Job—and the sufferings of Larry Browning. God's sovereignty is a big lesson. He has the right to do whatever He wants for whatever purpose He wants. He also has the right not to share that purpose with us.

The biggest lesson for me is how the power of God can sustain believers throughout the worst circumstances. For Job, it was the power to resist cursing God. For Larry, it's the power to maintain an ironclad faith throughout years of awful physical health.

The three of us continue to sit at the table and chat for several more minutes. Eventually we mosey out of the restaurant. I load Larry into the van and check the time. We were in the restaurant for over three hours. As we drive home, I glance at him. He's wide awake, relaxed, at ease. I think he enjoyed himself this morning.

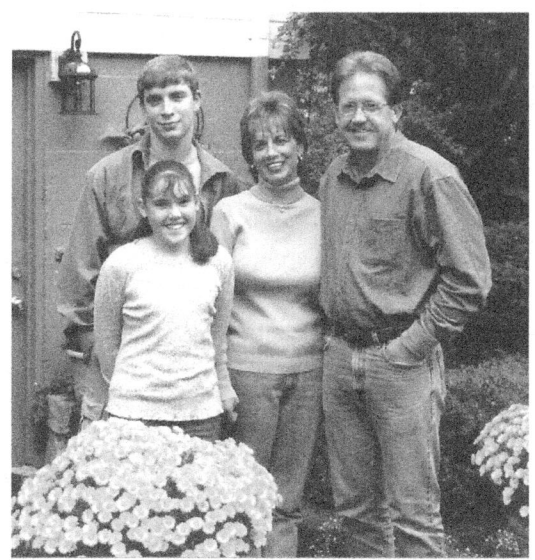
Family photo, October 2001

୫୦୧୫

15
THE HOPE

Larry is in the fourth day of an awakening, a reemergence from a semiconscious state. This morning he's alert, responsive, answering questions with a yes or no, eating and drinking.

The recent upturn is a far cry from a week ago, when he slept almost constantly, and barely ate or drank. He had difficulty taking meds by mouth, so the VA provided a topical form of Baclofen (which prevents involuntary muscle contractions) that absorbs into the skin. They also provided a liquid pain medication to be taken under the tongue. In his few waking moments last week, Larry rarely responded to questions. He seemed to be somewhere else.

But now he's back and I'm glad for it. My job is difficult when Larry is out of it; I'm extra tense and tend to make more mistakes. Much of the stress occurs when he doesn't eat or drink. I pray and start racking my brain for any way to get him to suck on the straw or take in a little applesauce. When he finally drinks and eats, I breathe a sigh of relief. And during those times, such as now, when he returns to consciousness, I smile.

These ups and downs of near-death and reemergence are especially anguishing for Ann. Despite the emotional ups and downs, she stays amazingly strong.

Ann is away doing errands and I'm alone with Larry in the kitchen, feeding him slices of fresh peach. He's nursing his second cup of coffee and I'm sipping from a mug of my own.

"I'm curious, Larry. What do you think about during those times we can't wake you up? It's like you're in a coma. Are you thinking about anything?"

He musters up some breath. "Yeah."

"I hope they're good thoughts. Are you learning things from the Lord during those times?"

"Yeah."

"So," I tease, "are you having out-of-body experiences like the apostle Paul and visiting the third heaven?" I'm thinking of 2 Corinthians 12:2-4.

He smiles.

"Is God teaching you things that you're not allowed to tell us?"

"Yeah."

I suspect he's joking and feed him the last slice of peach. Maybe he's not joking.

"Are you serious? Is God really teaching you things

you're not allowed to tell us?"

"Yes," he says straight-faced.

I wonder if he's mindlessly answering yes to every question.

"Would you like an English muffin?"

He pauses for breath. "No."

⋈⋊

Larry's bedtime routine requires Ann or another caregiver to maneuver him into a hammock-like sling which attaches to a hydraulic lift called a Hoyer. The crane-like apparatus lifts Larry out of his wheelchair and into his bed. The sling is then removed, the covers pulled over him, and the pillow positioned just right under his head. Ann kisses him goodnight.

Then he prays and his thoughts turn to heaven.

"I think about heaven all the time," he says, "especially at night when I go to bed. I'll often pray for God to heal me, or if He's not going to heal me physically, that He would just allow me to go home and be with Him."

Larry dreams nearly every night. They're often of the bizarre, nonsensical variety blamed on too much pizza, so there's probably no grand symbolic meaning hidden within them.

One thing stands out, though—he's only had one dream where he's in a wheelchair. "All the other dreams I'm physically able to do whatever I want."

Larry's beliefs about heaven are the same today as before he contracted MS. But if he still preached regularly, he says more of his sermons would be about heaven.

In July of 2010, Larry gave a message to a roomful of largely homeless men at the Eugene Mission. Being blind, he had to deliver the message without notes. He prepared by first listening to an audio reading of the gospel of John, chapter 14. Then, he organized the message inside his head. The following is an excerpt from Larry's presentation that night:

"Jesus was talking to his disciples [in John 14], but he was really talking to everyone who comes to Him to be their Savior and Lord. 'In my Father's house are many rooms. If it were not so, I would have told you. I go and prepare a place for you. And if I go, I'll come again and I'll take you where I am.' And Thomas, who was always known as the doubter, said, 'But Lord, we don't know where you're going, so how do we know how to get there?' Jesus said to Thomas, 'I am the way, the truth, and the life. No one comes to the Father, but through me.'

"We know that wherever Jesus was going, He was preparing a place for us, that when we pass from this life to the next, we'd be with Him. I've tried to imagine what heaven is like. I've looked around at this world, which God created, and I saw the beauty. But I also know that heaven will not be like this world and that it will not be filled with all kinds of hate and violence, bitterness, death, and destruction—all those things.

"There're only a few passages of scripture that we've been given that give us a glimpse into heaven. The apostle Paul wrote to the church at Corinth and said, 'No eye has seen, no ear has heard, no mind has conceived what God has prepared for those who love Him.' Also, in the book of Revelation, it talks about the new heaven and the new earth. There'll be no more tears; there'll be no more sorrow, no more pain. There'll be no more wheelchairs; there'll be no more hopelessness. There'll be no more economic downturns. There'll be no more struggles to find a job. Everything that causes us trouble in this life will pass away."

Larry's favorite hymn is, *What a Day That Will Be*. It describes how heaven will be free of illness, sorrows, hardship, pain and separations from loved ones.

Larry looks forward to the reunions celebrated in Heaven. Certainly he longs for his perfect resurrection body, but it's the relationships he anticipates the most.

"Being in the presence of God—I can't even imagine what it will be like when I actually see God for the first time and see the One who created everything. Then I think about the many people that I've known, members of the churches that I've pastored, my dad, my first wife Karen, just a lot of people who have preceded me in death. I think my favorite activity will be visiting with the people of my past, the Bible people—and having the opportunity just to spend the day with Jesus all by myself."

Larry mentions another great thing about heaven. "John MacArthur said the one thing that he's looking forward to in heaven is that there'll be no more sin. That's pretty hard to imagine."

Larry's temptations occur more in his mind than in his physical flesh. For example, he may be tempted to wallow in self-pity. He admits to succumbing to occasional pity parties, but he soon reorients his thinking heavenward.

Larry believes people would be better off if they were more heavenly-minded. The things of this world can easily become our main focus. But they can be stripped away in a moment—or over the course of ten years.

"I think for the most part we're too earthly-minded," he says. "It's hard for a lot of people to be heavenly-minded because they're caught up in wanting to enjoy life down here. Jesus said we are to fix our thoughts on heaven. I've heard it said that some people are so heavenly-minded that they're no earthly good; and some are so earthly-minded that they're no heavenly good. But I think the latter is probably more true. The circumstance I'm in now has certainly made me more heavenly-minded."

This is a hard truth to embrace—that trials and hardship can make us more heavenly minded. But it makes sense. If there's no likelihood for comfort or relief in this world, then our best hope comes by looking heavenward. Other alternatives exist, such as assisted suicide. But Larry rejects that option.

He finds hope and strength in Hebrews 12:2, "...looking to Jesus, the founder and perfecter of our faith, who for the joy that was set before him endured the cross, despising the shame, and is seated at the right hand of the throne of God."

Heaven is that joy.

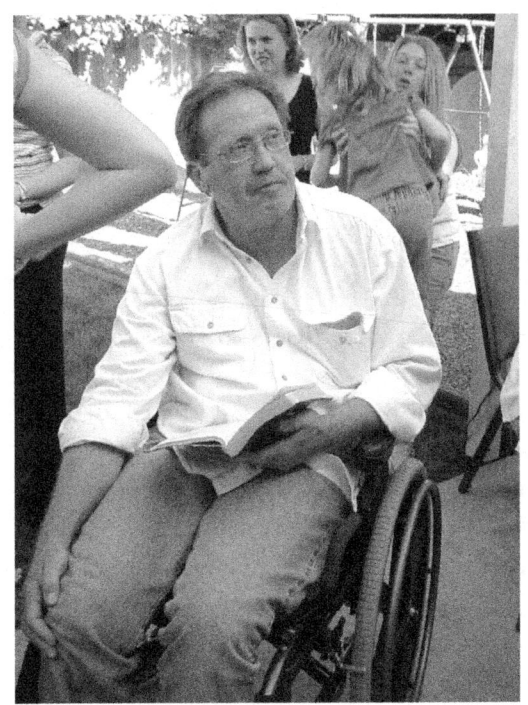

A role model? Absolutely. May 2004

ಌಂಡ

16
A BEACON

Larry believes strongly in the truth of Romans 8:28, "And we know that God causes all things to work together for good to those who love God, to those who are called according to His purpose." But the burden of quadriplegia never lets up; and there are days when Larry finds it difficult to recognize the good that comes from this.

During times of discouragement, he sometimes sees himself as a "spectacle" who draws a variety of responses from people. They respond with curiosity, shock, pity, queasiness, avoidance—or *comparative thinking*.

His ministry at the Eugene Mission inspired the spectacle idea. Says Larry, "It's kind of like, 'If you think you got it bad, look at Larry. So you're homeless and without work—you know, things could be worse.'"

Larry dislikes being used as an illustration of a worse-case scenario. But at the same time he acknowledges that the comparison can spur positive change in people. "Yeah, I think it's good for us to realize that our problems aren't nearly as insurmountable as other people's. I hear about people with problems that are far worse than mine."

Larry's uncomplaining attitude is a great example for someone such as myself who is tempted to grumble about trivial annoyances. It's a good thing for me to weigh my small problems against Larry's severe disability. He inspires me not to complain.

However, comparative thinking can yield negative results, such as pride and irresponsibility. One might think: *I'm sure glad I'm not as bad off as that guy. I'd rather forget about him and go have fun instead.*

Or, a healthy person may be preoccupied with a disability, blinding them to the fact that the guy in the wheelchair is a red-blooded human being with thoughts and feelings.

Also, well-intentioned healthy folks often focus attention on those who are "most visibly" worst off, neglecting others with seemingly lesser problems. For example, we might overlook someone on the verge of suicide, who, on the surface, appears to be doing okay.

So, Larry occasionally gets discouraged over his "spectacle" status.

"But that's just the human side of me that feels that way," says Larry, "because the scripture is real clear that God causes all things to work together for the good. So I know He has a purpose and a plan in mind. I'm required to walk by faith and not by sight. But sometimes you want to see Jesus with flesh on Him, you know. It would be nice to have God verbally speak or send an angel or something—kind of fill you in on what's going on. But I don't know if that happens. At least in my case it hasn't."

Let's be honest: Larry and others with disabilities are often viewed as spectacles. For example, a child's natural tendency is to stare at a disabled person out of curiosity. And when healthy adults notice severely disabled people, they tend to shake their heads and say, "How horrible—I hope that doesn't happen to me or my loved ones." Being repulsed or reacting in the extreme only creates walls between the healthy person and the disabled person. One must get over it.

When we view a fellow human being as a spectacle, we devalue him, dehumanize him, and forfeit opportunities to help and to learn. When the Larrys of this world attract our notice, our response can determine whether they are troubling objects or blessings to us from God.

Jerry Sittser, in his aforementioned book, *A Grace Disguised,* wrote a chapter titled *Whose Loss is Worse?* He feels it's a mistake to compare the severity of one loss to another. Sittser concludes, "The right question to ask is not, 'Whose is worse?' It is to ask, 'What meaning can be gained from suffering, and how can we grow through suffering?'"

And for myself, how can I grow and learn from a friend who is suffering? I think it begins with forming a correct view of my friend, recognizing our mutual humanity, and squarely facing his loss for what it is.

Larry grabs my attention, not as a spectacle, but as a beacon. He's like a bright, guiding light, a navigational aid. A beacon draws our notice for a purpose, sometimes to warn us of danger, other times to help us find the right course. We can choose to either follow the beacon into safe waters, or ignore it and crash our ship into the rocks.

Says Paige of her father, "I know he doesn't see it sometimes and it's hard for him, but I've seen how people's lives have been changed, because they see Christ in that chair. And they see God through him. He doesn't have anything left to give, but Christ still works through him and it's incredible. It's just incredible."

Ryan says this of his father: "He taught me how to be a man. Until Larry came into my life, I had no real male role-model. I had a very poor opinion of adult males because of what my biological father did. Larry was an example of what a man should be like, both spiritually and otherwise. There were a lot of little things that might seem insignificant to other people, but meant a lot to me. More than anything, he displayed Christ in his actions and attitudes. He also made me realize that godly men could be 'manly'"

଼ଠଔ

Many wonderful people have crossed my path, but my big brother Larry tops the list. He's the greatest hero of my life and a true example of what it means to be like Jesus. When I picture Larry in his wheelchair in the front row at church, it's as if the Lord is saying, "Study My servant, Larry. Reflect on his life, his words and his sufferings. Learn from him."

There are many lessons we can learn from the life, tribulations, and words of James Larry Browning. Here are some of the lessons I've learned from him:

> *"But a Samaritan, as he journeyed, came to where he* [a robbed, beaten man left for dead] *was, and when he saw him, he had compassion. He went to him and bound up his wounds, pouring on oil and wine. Then he set him on his own animal and brought him to an inn and took care of him." (Luke 10:33-34 ESV)*

Hoping to hear something deep and spiritual, I asked Larry, "What has your illness taught you? Has being confined to a wheelchair taught you things you wouldn't have learned otherwise?"

Larry threw the ball back at me (and you) with his answer, "Certainly it's taught me that the world knows little about wheelchair accessibility. And that's not spiritual; but it also knows very little about handicapped rooms in motels. It's also taught me that people generally are unaware of people in wheelchairs."

The story of the good Samaritan is more a call to action than a lesson. During his healthy years as a Christian, Larry cultivated a servant's heart. He was the good Samaritan. But as his disease progressed, he became the robbed, beaten man, so to speak. In his need, Larry provided opportunities for others to be good Samaritans. Some passed him by, others stopped and helped.

> *"Christ Jesus came into the world to save sinners, of whom I am the foremost. But I received mercy for this reason, that in me, as the foremost, Jesus Christ might display his perfect patience as an example to those who were to believe in him for eternal life." (1 Timothy 1:15-16 ESV)*

Before his conversion, the apostle Paul orchestrated

intense persecutions of the early Christian church and condoned the stoning of Stephen in Acts 8:1. God singles out "foremost" sinners and redeems them to show His patience and mercy. Make no mistake, sin damages both the sinner and those he or she sins against.

During the 1970's, Larry showed us what *not* to do. He chose to walk in the flesh and ignore the Holy Spirit's leading in his life. He believes he missed out on God's perfect will because of that period of rebellion. Addiction and a near-divorce are just a few bad results of those fleshly years.

However, the Lord causes *all* things, including past sins, to work for the good in the lives of those who love Him. Larry's wild years are a key part of a dramatic redemption story. As Paul wrote in 1 Corinthians 1:28-29 (ESV), "God chose what is low and despised in the world, even things that are not, to bring to nothing things that are, so that no human being might boast in the presence of God." This verse may perplex self-righteous types; however, it should give hope to those who feel trapped in sin. Lost sinners can look at Larry's life and say, "Wow, if God can save someone as bad as Larry and transform him into a productive man of God, then He can do the same for me."

"Jesus answered him, 'Truly, truly, I say to you, unless one is born again he cannot see the kingdom of God.'" (John 3:3 ESV)

At the age of seven, Larry made the best decision of his life. In tears, he asked Jesus Christ to be his Lord and Savior. The Holy Spirit responded to that prayer and entered Larry's heart. He experienced the new birth.

If you haven't been born again, Larry can tell you how: "First of all, you need to recognize that you are separated from Christ because of your sins and that God sent His son Jesus Christ to pay the debt for your sins. He did that on the cross. You couldn't pay the debt yourself, because God's standard is perfection and the only perfect person that could pay the debt was Jesus. So you need to acknowledge that you are a sinner and be willing to confess your sins, ask God's forgiveness, and then accept what God did for you through His son on the cross. Then be willing to surrender your life, to commit your life to God. Instead of saying, 'I'm gonna do it my way,' you say, 'I'm going to do it God's way.'"

"You will seek me and find me, when you seek me with all your heart." (Jeremiah 29:13 ESV)

In 1980, after ten years of roguish living, Larry began seeking God again. The bad habits didn't go away instantly. For two years, Larry tried to quit smoking pot and failed repeatedly. But he kept seeking God, confessing sin, asking for deliverance. Then one day in 1982, the desire for marijuana and tobacco vanished. Larry doesn't know why God chose that particular moment to deliver him. The timing was perfect, though. The miracle sparked a personal revival of service to God that has lasted to this day.

"Your word is a lamp to my feet and a light to my path." (Psalm 119:105 ESV)

For several months after God delivered him from addiction, Larry read and studied the Bible for two to three hours per day. His love and reverence for God's Word continues to the present. Larry now listens to an audio Bible on CD.

"Give thanks to the Lord, for he is good, for his steadfast love endures forever." (Psalm 136:1 ESV)

Over and over throughout the Psalms, we are told to give

thanks to the Lord. People with selfish tendencies (who, me?) find it difficult to offer God thanks. When we pray, our natural inclination is to ask God for what we don't have, rather than to thank Him for what He's already given us.

Says Larry, "God has taught me to be more appreciative of the things I have and to not take them for granted, because He has blessed me tremendously."

"But who are you, O man, to answer back to God? Will what is molded say to its molder, 'Why have you made me like this?'" (Romans 9:20 ESV)

Larry believes strongly in the sovereignty of God. The Lord can do whatever He wants with His creation. "The bottom line," says Larry, "is that He desires to be glorified through my life. He wants me to have the attitude and the mindset that would bring glory to Him, to give testimony to the goodness of God despite my condition and to the grace of God that He gives me each day to live in this condition. Ultimately, God is the potter and we are the clay and He can do whatever He wants with us. As Job discovered, he really had no grounds for questioning what God does. Although I don't know the specifics of why God allows me to be in this condition, I know that the ultimate purpose is to glorify Him."

"...looking to Jesus, the founder and perfecter of our faith, who for the joy that was set before him endured the cross...." (Hebrews 12:2 ESV)

When asked to give principles that help him through the day, Larry answered, "When my mind is fixed on God, it's not fixed on me and my condition. It's fixed on God and His purposes. Also, I fix my eyes on Jesus because I think of all that He endured on my behalf—but He also endured it for the joy that was set before Him. So the principal is that I fix my eyes on Jesus and I also think about what lies ahead. This is a temporal state of being, but one day I will be completely whole—and that will be eternal."

"And all who believed were together and had all things in common." (Acts 3:44 ESV)

Larry loves his fellow believers—and likes to be around them. He promotes unity within the body of Christ without compromising Biblical truth. When he entered his first pastorate, he encountered a congregation that had split over a petty issue. Through prayer, patience and love, Larry helped unify the members and get their focus on their loving heavenly Father.

"Rather, speaking the truth in love, we are to grow up in every way into him who is the head, into Christ…" (Ephesians 4:15 ESV)

In this postmodern world where Biblical truth is marginalized (even within the evangelical church), Larry is unafraid to proclaim the great doctrines of the Bible. If he still preached regularly, he'd emphasize them even more.

"The reason I would preach more doctrinal messages is because too many Christians don't even know what they believe." Would he thump people's heads with his Bible? See the next lesson for the answer.

"Love your neighbor as yourself." (Matthew 22:39 NIV)

Larry practices what he preaches. As a pastor, he taught the truth on Sunday and loved people all seven days of the week. Whether it was chopping wood for an elderly widow at the Dorris church, or ensuring that everybody at the Spokane church received at least an offer of help from a deacon, Larry lived to serve and meet people's needs.

"I was sick and you looked after me, I was in prison and you came to visit me." (Matthew 25:36 NIV)

Larry visited the sick while sick himself. He visited prisoners, knowing full well his past drug dealings should have landed him in the slammer. All of us are sinners, deserving the wrath of God. Yet God showed us mercy by sending His Son to bear our sins. We in turn reflect God's mercy by visiting prisoners. Larry went the extra mile and put together care packages for inmates, using his own money. He followed Christ's example of meeting the physical needs of people, as well as their spiritual needs.

"Blessed are those who mourn, for they shall be comforted." (Matthew 5:4 ESV)

The losses of his first wife, Karen, and his father, were huge blows to Larry. Eventually he found comfort and healing. The Lord used those tragedies to give Larry a heart of compassion for others who have suffered loss.

As a pastor, Larry felt honored "…when people invited me into really hard times." He tells of a senior woman from his church, who asked him to sit with her by her husband's bedside as he passed away. Larry views that as one of the greatest honors of his life, that she would invite him to join her in those final moments.

"Humble yourselves, therefore, under God's mighty hand, that he may lift you up in due time." (1 Peter 5:6 NIV)

Says Larry, "He [God] is also teaching me humility, because it's a very humbling experience when you can't do anything—and literally everything has to be done for you."

"If anyone would come after me, let him deny himself and take up his cross daily and follow me. For whoever would save his life will lose it, but whoever loses his life for my sake will save it." (Luke 9:23 ESV)

For the ten-plus years of his illness, Larry has been forced to die to himself through each stage of decline. Some sacrifices hurt more than others. Giving up his pastorate meant dying to his calling, his purpose, his passion.

Says Paige, "The thing that broke my heart the most was that he was giving up what God had called him to do. I know for him that was the hardest thing he's ever had to do."

Larry has mentioned several times that his loss of sight is one of the biggest blows. Blindness has made him realize the importance of eyesight for good communication. The inability to see facial expressions or other non-verbal cues creates a serious communication barrier—and relationships have always been top priority with him.

"Indeed, I count everything as loss because of the surpassing worth of knowing Christ Jesus my Lord. For his sake I have suffered the loss of all things and count them as rubbish, in order that I may gain Christ...." (Philippians 3:8 ESV)

Larry's family has suffered incredible heartache during his illness. How have they responded?

Says Paige, "This disease has strengthened all of our faith—my mom, my brother, my dad and me. As hard as it is to say, if this is what it took for us to be where we are now, it was worth it. But no matter what happens, it's not your life to live, it's God's. God is your Father and He will take care of you, and He has. Don't ever lose your faith, because it is what will get you through everything."

Says Ryan about his father, "His faith was very genuine

and strong. The most notable part was how it only got stronger with his illness."

"My grace is sufficient for you, for my power is made perfect in weakness." (2 Corinthians 12:9 ESV)

One of the greatest lessons I've learned from working with Larry is that no matter how bad circumstances get in our lives, God's power will sustain us. For Job, it was the power to resist cursing God. For Larry, it's the power to remain faithful without becoming bitter. He offers the following advice for receiving spiritual strength: "We need to yield to the Holy Spirit, recognize our weakness, and as Paul said, we need to die daily, put off our selfish ambitions and trust the Lord."

"You keep him in perfect peace whose mind is stayed on you, because he trusts in you." (Isaiah 26:3 ESV)

When asked if he feels God's peace in his heart, Larry answers, "Yeah, when I stay focused on Him, I do. When I get myself focused on my problems, I lose God's peace. I think the key is to keep focused on God and the promises that deal with the eternal, or things to come, rather than the temporal."

"Be still, and know that I am God. I will be exalted among the nations, I will be exalted in the earth." (Psalm 46:10 ESV)

Says Larry, "God has taught me the importance of being still and waiting on Him. He's kind of put me in a position where I really don't have any other choice. But also, at the same time I've learned that although I'm confined in this wheelchair, I'm not confined in my usefulness to God. I spend a great deal more time in prayer—praying for lost people, praying for my family, praying for other needs that I've been made aware of."

"I have learned the secret of being content in any and every situation, whether well fed or hungry, whether living in plenty or in want. I can do everything through him who gives me strength." (Philippians 4:12-13 NIV)

Many people watch TV for hours, overeat, spend much of their free (or work) time on electronic or social media, get drunk, gamble, take drugs and stay overly busy—all for the purpose of masking their discontentment. Larry doesn't have those options, yet he's learned to be content. Says Larry, "He [God] puts you in circumstances where you can either learn contentment or not. It's kind of like an exercise on building your faith."

"My desire is to depart and be with Christ, for that is far better. But to remain in the flesh is more necessary on your account." (Philippians 1:23-24 ESV)

As Larry enters the final phase of his earthly life, he's unable to talk, except for an occasional whisper of "yes" or "no." His church family feels antsy, uncomfortable, unsure of what to do. More and more, the prayers have become something like, "Lord, don't let him suffer any more. Please take him soon." I've said that prayer too, because Larry would be so much happier in heaven. But God is sovereign and will take him at the precise moment He wants to take him. The Lord has a purpose for prolonging Larry's life beyond what seems reasonable to us. Each day that Larry remains in the flesh is necessary on our account. Lately I've prayed, "Dear God, show me what I can learn from a quadriplegic blind man who can't speak."

"The Spirit himself bears witness with our spirit that we are children of God, and if children, then heirs—heirs of God and fellow heirs with Christ...." (Romans 8:16-17 ESV)

Writer Lyla Swafford suffers from cerebral palsy and can often be seen at Oregon Christian Writers conferences, riding on a blue scooter. In Marion Duckworth's article *Lyla Swafford: It Takes More than Legs to Stand* (Oregon Christian Writers Newsletter, Winter 2012), Lyla explains how her self-worth reached a low point as she pursued a career following graduation from George Fox College (now George Fox University). "…when the doors to a career were slammed in my face, disappointment and disillusionment overwhelmed me. So my walk with God became as precarious as my gait and balance. But He was setting the stage for me to learn that my value comes from my relationship with Him and not from what I do."

Christians are God's adopted children and fellow heirs with Christ. This lofty title is given by grace, through faith. We don't earn it through performance.

What can I learn from a quadriplegic blind man who can't speak? Larry's worth is immense, not based on what he does or says, but on who he is in Christ. All believers partake in this elevated status. There's no room for pride, however, since it's entirely a gift from God.

"These were commended for their faith, yet none of them received what had been promised." (Hebrews 11:39 NIV)

Larry has maintained great faith, though it appears he will not be rewarded in *this* life. Says Ryan of his father, "By watching how his faith got stronger and stronger as his condition got worse and worse, he showed me what it means to continue to praise God in any situation. He also showed me what it meant to trust God with every aspect of my life."

Says Paige, "Dad has been faced with ten years of something that's incredibly hard, and yet he's still chosen to be faithful to God. I've never heard him once blame God for what has happened to him. There's so much crud out there in terms of Christianity and different views. His faith is the faith of the Bible. That's where he finds his strength. It's one of the purest faiths I've ever seen."

"Give, and it shall be given unto you; good measure, pressed down, and shaken together, and running over, shall men give into your bosom." (Luke 6:38 KJV)

Larry is not a "name it, claim it" kind of guy, but he does believe the Lord wants us to tithe, to give one tenth of our gross income to the church. Larry and Ann give additional money, over and above the tithe, to missionaries and other Christian organizations. They believe the Lord blesses those who give generously. Over the years, God has been faithful to meet the Brownings' financial needs.

"I have become all things to all people, that by all means I might save some." (1 Corinthians 9:22 ESV)

Thanks to his diverse past, Larry can relate to a wide variety of people. One of the biggest obstacles for me when I first started working for Larry was a concern that I would never be able to relate to or empathize with him because of his illness. Perhaps I viewed him as a spectacle and allowed that to blind me to his humanity. To my surprise, I found that it wasn't necessary for me to deeply understand his disability in order to cultivate a good friendship with him. Larry has said, "Being handicapped is something that—until you've experienced it—you really know little about it. I never would have been able to relate to someone in a wheelchair without having been in one myself."

Though I can't identify with Larry's disability, we both share the same humanity—and the same Lord. We can fellowship and be friends. On the other hand, a basic understanding of his disability is needed so I can provide adequate assistance. And it's good to be sensitive to what *not* to say, such as not greeting him with a thoughtless, "How ya doing, Larry?"

"Do everything without complaining...." (Philippians 2:14 NIV)

I've never heard Larry complain. If someone asks about his illness, he will matter-of-factly describe some of his difficulties. If he needs something to alleviate discomfort or pain, he will let you know. But he chooses not to fish for sympathy or pity. Instead, he'll look outside of himself and ask what's happening in *your* life.

"...much more in my absence, work out your own salvation with fear and trembling, for it is God who works in you, both to will and to work for his good pleasure." (Philippians 2:12-13 ESV)

The apostle Paul was a great teacher, but eventually he had to resume his travels and trust God to transform the church at Philippi. A significant lesson I learned by working with Larry is, at the end of the day, my sanctification (spiritual growth) is a process that happens between God and me. When God delivered Larry from marijuana and tobacco addictions, it wasn't due to his wife's vehement admonitions for him to quit. She didn't change Larry; the Holy Spirit did. Likewise, Larry is not the Holy Spirit in my life. He's an amazing guy and I've learned much from him, but he cannot change me. People may inspire me, but my human enthusiasm eventually wanes. We can learn much from others, but applying the lessons takes the power of the Holy Spirit.

Larry's final sermon as pastor at Valley Hills focused less on sentimentality and more on the Christian's active responsibility. He told his congregation, "When I stand before God, I will give an account of my work at Valley Hills. Whether it was in vain or not will be the proof of your lives, of how you lived out your life—if you continue to live in obedience and harmony, if you continue to put feet to your faith, if you continue to shine as the lights that God called you to."

Larry enjoyed good movies and loved watching sports. He liked reading and hearing a good story; and he would hope this book touches your hearts. But my guess is he wouldn't want people to limit themselves to a fleeting emotional experience. He'd hope that readers learn something from his story and, with God's help, apply it to their lives.

If you are an unbeliever, the first "application" would be for you to pray and ask Jesus to be your Lord and Savior.

For believers—that you grow in your relationship with Christ, love God and glorify Him. When asked to explain the meaning of life, Larry said, "I think the meaning of life is to know God and bring glory to Him. It's all about God; it's not about us."

The poem, *Footprints in the Sand,* describes how the narrator dreams about walking through life with the Lord by his/her side. This results in two sets of footprints in the sand. During especially hard times, only one set of footprints is seen, and the narrator assumes God has left. He/she feels abandoned by God during these periods, but the Lord says, "The times when you have seen only one set of footprints is when I carried you."

As I write these words, Larry's breaths become fainter and fainter. He struggles to even say yes or no. Two days ago, I asked him if he's felt God's presence more in the last few weeks.

He raised his eyebrows and said clearly, "Yes." I asked if he's experiencing more of the Lord's peace. "Yes."

Larry does appear to be at peace. Ann's noticed it too.

I think Jesus is carrying him now. Larry's time with us is nearly complete and his glimpses of heaven are clearer than ever. Soon, he will see the face of God—and the confines of this world will be gone forever.

AFTERWORD

I push open the stubborn, spring-loaded door to the Vida Café and a bell jingles overhead. The door thuds behind me, bruising the nose of Jack Frost, who's banished outside on this chilly January morning, 2012. Fresh snow blankets the nearby McKenzie valley hills. I'm looking forward to a hot cup of coffee, the café's killer Denver omelet, and a cozy time perusing the newspaper.

I take a seat at a table in the center of the small restaurant and glance at the menu. A waitress, wearing trendy, black-framed rectangular glasses, takes my order, then heads to the kitchen. She returns with my coffee. I open the newspaper.

The door jingles and a cute, petite, twenty-something brunette enters.

"Are you still serving breakfast?" she asks the waitress.

"Yes."

The young woman exits the café.

A minute or two passes and I look outside. A young man in an electric wheelchair rolls across the parking lot. He operates the control toggle with his right hand. The petite brunette walks ahead of him and pushes against the resistant entrance. Her brow furrows as the door slowly gives. She holds it open for the guy in the wheelchair.

He drives up the concrete ramp. The wheels stall against the bulky threshold. She vainly attempts to pull the wheelchair inside with one hand, while holding the door open with the other.

I hop to my feet and hustle toward them.

"Can I help?" I ask, and hold the door open.

She nods, moves behind the wheelchair, and pushes on the handles with both hands. The pair make it past the threshold and I keep the door open as they squeeze by me.

"Thank you," she says.

"You bet." I sit back down. My breakfast arrives.

They choose a corner booth and he maneuvers his wheelchair alongside the end of the table. She sits near him. They're in my line of sight, and I allow occasional stealthy glances in their direction.

He's a dark-haired, handsome fellow, maybe late twenties. He looks tough, like a warrior. I could imagine him a casualty of the Afghanistan or Iraq War. His fingers move, but his forearms stay fixed on the armrests.

Lord, I hope he can feed himself.

They order their food. A few minutes pass and their breakfast arrives.

She begins to feed him.

My eyes tear up. I look down at the newspaper and ask God to keep me from sobbing. I pray that the young man doesn't notice my red, watery eyes. Undoubtedly, the couple has already experienced a lifetime of drama; they don't need more from me.

I try to focus on the news, but my mind wanders. At least the omelet tastes good. It takes more than sadness to ruin my appetite.

They finish eating and move to pay their bill. He drives the wheelchair past my table and says, "Thanks for opening the door."

I nod.

Exiting is easier for them because the threshold is lower from the inside. She pulls the door open and holds it. He drives out without a hitch.

I pay my bill, exit the café and enter my pickup. I pull onto the highway. No one can see me. Now the sobs come.

My big brother Larry, the greatest hero of my life, passed away two months ago.

I'm relieved that he experiences utter bliss in heaven, but tribulations continue in the world he left behind. The couple seemed upbeat in the café, chatting about day-to-day things. But I know they experience hardship on a daily basis. I pray that God would bless them, soften their pain and somehow bring seasons of happiness into their lives.

ꝏ

As Larry neared the end, both his breathing and ability to swallow had diminished to practically nothing. He was no longer conscious. In the hours after midnight on November 5, 2011, his lungs had accumulated enough fluid that the hospice nurse felt death was imminent.

An all-night vigil began. By his bedside in the final moments were Ann, Ryan, Ryan's wife Rebecca, Ann's brother Dave, weekend caregiver Ray, and RN/neighbor Lisa. Paige was in Riverside, California, over nine hundred miles away. Miss Kitty slept in her usual position on Larry's lap. Ray read aloud from the Psalms.

Larry took his final breath at 11:05 AM. Ray had just finished Psalm 20:7. "Some trust in chariots and some in horses, but we trust in the name of the Lord our God."

The verse fit, with its war imagery of chariots and horses. Throughout his life, Larry's physical, spiritual and mental battles were overwhelming, especially during his last ten years.

He fought and won by placing his complete trust in the Lord his God, who fortified him with inner strength to endure onslaughts of intense, prolonged tribulation.

And yet, in the midst of the battles, Larry reflected God's peace.

The war is over. The pain is gone. Larry's spirit is alive,

ecstatic—and eternally free from that coffin-like body.

His body was laid to rest at Springfield Memorial Gardens Cemetery, where his father Jay, first wife Karen, and close friend Tim Ownbey were buried. His memorial service took place on Veterans Day at McKenzie Bible Fellowship. About three hundred attended.

Pastor Dick Roberts officiated and gave a clear presentation of the gospel, as Larry had requested. In a moving ceremony, a two-man color guard unfolded and displayed an American flag. They refolded the flag and presented it to Ann in honor of her husband's military service.

The memorial stirred me, but my sentiments were checked by a few nagging questions. In the days, months and years ahead, would Larry become just a faint recollection in the minds of those who knew him? Would they be inspired by the memory or only sigh at the thought of Larry's disability? What lasting impact would his life have on them?

But those questions were based on my limited, human perspective, not on God's promises and sovereignty. Larry was a man of great faith. He believed that *all* of his life would be used by God for the good. In his introduction to this book, he wrote, "I saw how God uses all things, the bad as well as the good, to accomplish His purposes. Throughout my twenty years of pastoring, the truth of Romans 8:28 has been confirmed time and time again. Today as I sit in this wheelchair, physically unable to do anything, God continues to show me that He does work all things together for the good to those who *love Him* and are called according to *His purposes.*'"

This book could end with a sentimental statement about how great Larry was—and indeed he was a great man to those who knew him. But he wouldn't have wanted that. Larry knew that any good he possessed came from God, and that the Lord can do the same in you.

Physically, Larry was the weakest man I've ever known. Spiritually, he was a giant. He would be the first to say that his inner strength came from God. As the apostle Paul said, "For the sake of Christ, then, I am content with weaknesses, insults, hardships, persecutions, and calamities. For when I am weak, then I am strong." (2 Corinthians 12:10 ESV)

What are we to make of the life of James Larry Browning? He was a soldier, hippie, preacher, husband, widower, father, and a modern-day Job. But ultimately, he was a man who knew, loved and trusted God—and lovingly served the many people who entered his life.

In an April 2011 interview, Larry was asked to give advice to readers who struggle with hardship. He said, "I would just like to tell people that there's no easy solution to what they're going through, but if they have faith and trust in God and Jesus Christ, they have something to look forward to—to trust that God knows far better that we do. I think one of my favorite passages is in Proverbs 3:5-6. It says, 'Trust in the Lord with all your heart, don't lean on your own understanding. In all your ways acknowledge him, and he will direct your path.' I think that's a pretty good philosophy of life, and that's what I'd leave with people—put all your trust in God."

ཕༀ

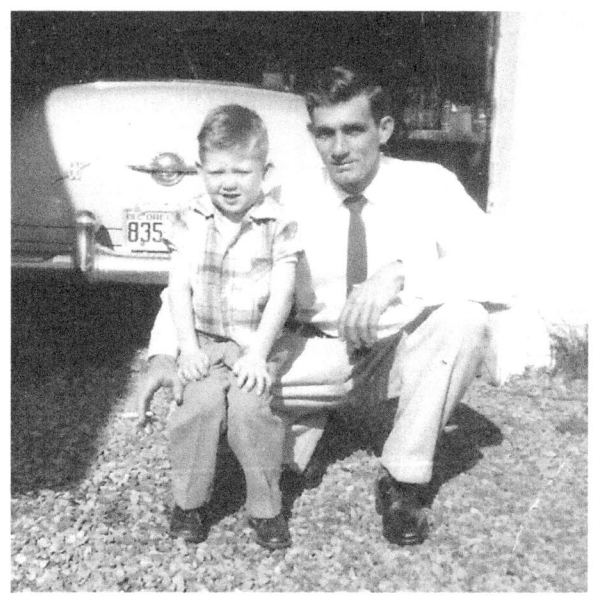

Larry and his father, Jay, about 1954

Made in the USA
Las Vegas, NV
02 October 2021